Healing from the Heart

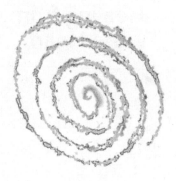

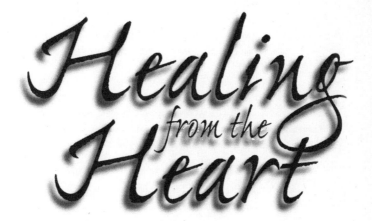

A Guide to Christian Healing
for Individuals and Groups

Rochelle Graham *Hands on Experience*

Traditions and Liturgies **Flora Litt**

Wayne Irwin *The Scientific Evidence*

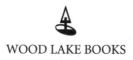

WOOD LAKE BOOKS

Editors: Jim Taylor, Dianne Greenslade
Cover design: Margaret Kyle
Interior design: Julie Bachewich
Cover photograph: Mike Swartzentruber
Consulting art director: Robert MacDonald

Unless otherwise noted, all biblical references are from the New Revised Standard Version.

AT WOOD LAKE BOOKS

we practice what we publish, guided by a concern for fairness, justice, and equal opportunity in all of our relationships with employees and customers.

Wood Lake Books Publishing Inc. is an employee-owned company, committed to caring for the environment and all creation. Wood Lake Books recycles, reuses and composts, and encourages readers to do the same. Resources are printed on recycled paper and more environmentally friendly groundwood papers (newsprint), whenever possible. The trees used are replaced through donations to the Scoutrees for Canada Program. Ten percent of all profit is donated to charitable organizations.

We acknowledge the financial support of the Government of Canada through the Book Publishing Industry Development Program for our publishing activities.

Canadian Cataloguing in Publication Data

Graham, Rochelle, 1953-
Healing from the heart

Includes bibliographical references and index.
ISBN 1-55145-294-4

1. Spiritual healing. 2. Spiritual healing—History of doctrines.
3. Health—Religious aspects—Christianity. I. Litt, Flora, 1929-
II. Irwin, Wayne, 1944- III. Taylor, Jim, 1941- IV. Title.
BT732.5.G72 1998   234'.131   C98-910273-4

Published by Wood Lake Books
Winfield, BC Canada

Printed in Canada by Transcontinental Printing Inc.
Peterborough, Ontario

Dedication

*Dedicated to the well-being
of you, the reader, and
those to whom you minister.*

Contents

Appendices

Acknowledgments

We wish to express our appreciation to family and friends for the support and encouragement they have given us in the writing of this book. We particularly wish to express our appreciation to Jim Taylor, our editor, who has worked patiently and lovingly with us.

Rochelle Graham
Flora Litt
Wayne Irwin

Editor's Preface

I am, by nature, a skeptic. I challenge anything taken for granted, and drive my friends wild by constantly testing their ideas in my mind to find the flaws, the weaknesses, the loopholes.

The first time I saw Rochelle Graham in action, at the Naramata Centre in BC in 1994, I had dozens of questions. We had gathered to see a demonstration of Healing Touch. The name seemed a bit of a misnomer, for Rochelle never touched the person she was demonstrating on. Her hands hovered a few inches from her subject, moving rather as if she were lovingly brushing Rapunzel's long silky hair.

During that demonstration, someone asked, "What are you trying to do here?"

The answer should have been something practical, something like, "I'm sensing an emotional knot in the left shoulder, and I'm trying to untangle it and ease the tension."

But from somewhere – and Rochelle insists that the words came unbidden, that she had no prior intention of uttering them – came the answer: "I want to change the church's mind about healing."

Four years later, Rochelle Graham, Flora Litt, and Wayne Irwin have teamed up to produce a book intended to do just that – to change the church's mind about healing. And it appeals to my still-skeptical mind. For it is not a compilation of miraculous cures, piled into an insurmountable mound of self-congratulation. Nor does it ask you to accept uncritically the traditions of some Oriental system of healing.

Granted, it does acknowledge insights from Eastern practices. But it also identifies insights from experimental science, and from the Bible, and from our heritage of Christian worship. The healing does not depend on the system or philosophy; rather, the system or philosophy supports the healing.

Let me explain that from my own experience. Years ago, before our son Stephen died of cystic fibrosis, he used to get blinding headaches at night. They were severe enough to make him nauseated, to make him whimper in pain, to leave him shivering helplessly. I discovered, by loving trial and error, that if I gently massaged certain places at the back of his skull, coupled with murmured suggestions to direct his chaotic thoughts, I could reduce the severity of the headache enough for him to go back to sleep. It's the same principle that leads mothers to stroke the heads of children who have a stomach ache, or to kiss it better when they've skinned their knees.

In my later years, I've discovered that I was practicing guided meditation – a healing technique that comes to us from Eastern religions. And the places I was massaging were, by coincidence, also points used in acupuncture, points that lie directly on some of the so-called "meridians" that extend through our bodies.

The healing that I did with Stephen – however temporary it was – did not depend on my subscribing to some exotic religion or belief. Rather, the exotic confirmed the rightness of what I had learned through my own experience.

So it is in this book. The three authors offer you their evidence. It's up to you to weigh it, to decide if it corroborates your own experience.

Although all three collaborated on the entire book, each took a lead role in writing specific chapters. Each of these tends to reflect the author's personal interests.

Rochelle's draws primarily on her own experience of healing. Rochelle works directly with people, one on one. Hers is a "hands on" narrative. Much of what she says is intended to encourage you to develop and practice your own capabilities for healing. Her credibility, I suspect, lies in her personality. Whether or not I believe in the theory of Healing Touch – and I have seen its effects on people close to me – I trust her.

I trust Flora Litt and Wayne Irwin too, in different ways.

Flora Litt's chapters focus on work with groups in the context of worship. Although both she and Wayne Irwin have been extensively involved in Therapeutic Touch, in these chapters she concentrates on the historic tradition of healing in the church. She recognizes that for most of us, the personal use of hands on healing may be more than we are ready for. But we can all participate in healing services, in prayer groups, in caring circles.

Flora helps us explore our rich Christian history of scripture and liturgy. She convinces me that healing is not a new-fangled fad, a trendy thing that explodes like fireworks in a summer night and then fades away, but a deep underlying current that has been part of our past and our present, even when we were unaware of it.

Wayne too has been conducting prayer and healing ministry in the United Church of Canada for 15 years, but for the purposes of this book, he directs our attention to the growing body of scientific evidence that supports healing. I particularly value his insights. In the Myers-Briggs typology for determining personality types, I am a strong "T" – a "thinker" who needs to understand things. Wayne has not assembled the kind of evidence usually presented to justify claims of "miraculous cures": before and after X rays showing that a tumor has vanished; dental charts documenting disappearing cavities; paraplegics getting up and walking… Such evidence may be overwhelming, but it is not convincing, because it fails to explain to me HOW such things can happen. Wayne has chosen, instead, to help me see the basis for the power of prayer, to recognize the reality of dimensions that go beyond our usual five senses.

I am not, myself, a "healer." I have no sense of power, or light, or strength, flowing through me into someone else. But I don't have to be a healer to believe in the reality of healing. And after working with Rochelle and Flora and Wayne, I am no longer as skeptical about its possibilities.

I hope that when you have read this book, you will not be skeptical either.

JIM TAYLOR

Many in the church today are suspicious of healing.
Some see various forms of healing as promotion of other beliefs and religions;
some see healing as manipulation and exploitation.
*The focus of this book, as **Rochelle Graham** explains, is Christian healing.*

1

Healing From the Heart

There is a great deal published today about healing, and about different methods or techniques of healing. Most of these writings are secular in their language and beliefs. There are many paths of healing present in the world today and present throughout many cultures and religious paths. In this book, however, our concern is Christian healing.

In his book *Healing and Christianity*, Morton Kelsey, an Episcopal priest, counselor, and author of over 20 books, describes one of the most characteristic aspects of Christian healers. It is, he says, their capacity to love, to be channels of divine love. Love is not unique to the Christian faith (or any faith for that matter) but our teacher did model a path that had love and compassion as the central core of his ministry. As Jesus said,

> *You shall love the Lord your God with all your heart,*
> *and with all your soul, and with all your mind.*
> *This is the greatest and the first commandment.*
> *And a second is like it: You shall love your neighbor as yourself.*
> (Matthew 22:37-39)

So clearly a Christian ministry is characterized by love – not an emotional infatuation, but a love that reflects its divine source, the quality of love that we see in Jesus Christ.

We know that much of Jesus' activity centered around healing. He sent his disciples – his closest friends and later others – out to perform this basic ministry. The followers of Jesus carried on his healing ministry. They believed that the same Spirit that had worked through him, worked through them when they healed in Jesus' name.

From the gospel records, it's clear that Jesus touched those he healed. The power went forth from him. He used different techniques depending on the problem, but always he reached out in compassion and love. He listened, and he restored relationships. The leper was made whole and clean and restored to the community.

Healings continue to happen today. Let me tell you about one of them.

Anne came to see me somewhat apprehensively. She had fibromyalgia, a disease causing severe muscle pain and stiffness. She had experienced this pain for eight years. It had limited her ability to be mobile and had severely curtailed her ability to enjoy life. At times when Anne was unable to get out of bed, her mother had to come to assist with the necessary household activities required by three children in the house.

As Anne described the pain to me, she said that her left side was worse than her right. As I talked with her, it was also clear that in this package called pain, there were physical problems such as thoracic outlet syndrome – pain caused by pressure on the nerves and blood vessels where they leave the neck and go into the arm – and emotional and spiritual pains.

I began to work with Anne, with the energy of her body. As I worked, I sensed that in spite of what Anne had told me, the left side of her body was actually feeling better than the right side. This puzzled me.

Anne smiled, " I guess I have to tell you." The night before, she had attended a healing service at the local Anglican church. She had specifically asked for healing for her left side. She described a man praying for her; during this time, she said, a profound white light had filled her left side, lifting the pain, the sadness, and the bitterness that accompanied her disability.

Anne then looked at me and shyly said, " I forgot to ask for my right side to be healed too."

What happened during the healing service? It would be hard to attribute the healing to Anne's faith, for this was her first time in a church for many years. She only went because her mother convinced her to try. Anne went as a skeptic but, perhaps in desperation, open to anything.

Anne believed that she was now on the road to getting well. I continued to work with her over the next few years. Life didn't get easier for Anne, but she received support to heal many aspects of her life, to renew herself spiritually, and to become strong at her broken places.

In carrying on the work started so long ago, we are called to be faithful to the path modeled by Jesus and the early Christians. Part of the faith of the early Christians was the belief that their God was a loving, compassionate, healing God who expected a healing ministry from Christian followers. We three authors – Flora, Wayne, and I – are deeply committed to the path of healing within the Church. Although we each have different backgrounds, we have in common a fundamental belief that God, revealed in Christ and acting by the Holy Spirit, works through us as we make ourselves available to facilitate healing.

What Is Health, Anyway?

In our culture, we tend to have a deep suspicion of anything unexplainable. We also tend to confuse "health" and "cure."

Despite working for over two hours to stabilize the woman's heart, the physician was unable to restore the normal heart rhythm. He called her children in to say goodbye. They entered the ward nervously, moving as if in one organic step, to embrace her, to assure her of their never-failing love. The moment they touched their mother, her heart rhythm changed from the potentially lethal rhythm of over 120 beats per minute to a normal rhythm. Half an hour later she was awake, talking with them and helping them arrange her bedding and her clothes.

There is no medical explanation for this change. Were the woman's own healing resources roused by feeling a connection with her family? Did her children influence her health by focusing healing energy upon her by their intimate touch? Was this "healing from the heart" ?

And what is health anyway? Jesus apparently defined it as "life in its fullness." He said,

> *I came that they may have life, and have it abundantly.*
> (John 10:10)

Dictionaries define health as freedom from illness, from disease, or as a state of normal and efficient functioning. Others describe health at the physical level as freedom from pain, a state of physical well-being; at the emotional level as freedom from passion, a dynamic state of serenity and calm; at the mental level as freedom from selfishness, a sense of total unification with truth.

A Sign of Wholeness

For this book, we three authors treat health as much more than freedom from illness or deliverance from disease, and certainly much more than a static condition of being. It is a fluid experience of wholeness, of balance and harmony. Health is a continuous process involving ongoing interplay between the physical, emotional, mental, spiritual, and relational aspects of the self. Health, as we intend it to be understood here, also extends beyond the individual to an interplay with the environment, the family, the social milieu, the national and global scene, and with nature itself. Every choice or lack of choice we make, every action or lack of action we take, whether in relation to our bodies or to our world, affects our health.

The Latin word *salvatio* from which comes our word "salvation," means "being made whole or sound." Likewise, the Greek word *sozo* can be interpreted as meaning "to save," "to heal," or "to make whole." The Hebrew word *shalom* has similar implications. *Shalom* is commonly used in Christian churches as a synonym for "peace" – true enough, if we understand "peace" to mean "total peace," a complete harmony of body and soul, person and environment.

"Health," then – "salvation" or "wholeness" – depends upon the well-being of every facet of our make-up. It depends on a constantly changing relationship between the physiology of the body and its interaction with our emotions, thoughts, and spirituality. Health cannot be understood apart from its context: the food we eat, the air we breathe, the land we live on, the climate we experience, the water that we drink, and the relationship within family and community.

For example, you can go to bed feeling healthy and peaceful, but through the night your life companion, who has a severe cold, coughs continually. You, consequently, have a restless night. You wake late, fatigued. To offset your weariness, you gulp an extra cup of coffee and skip breakfast. Both the caffeine and the lack of food adversely affect your physiology. On your way to work, you are further upset by an extended delay on the road because of an accident ahead; you arrive late for an important meeting. Obviously, your state of health is very different now from what it was 12 hours before.

The word "health" originated as the old Saxon word *hal* from which we also get the words "hale," "whole," and even "hello." When we greet someone "Hello," or ask "How are you?" we are asking after their health.

Wholeness implies many parts. Our physical bodies have many parts; we are beings of many emotions, thoughts and relationships. We are part of a family, a community, a world where we humans are only one part of the whole.

Holistic health recognizes this interaction among the parts of the whole being. The emphasis is on the whole person, the balance within, the balance and harmony in how an individual interacts with family and friends, the environment, their community and their God. It also recognizes both past and present interactions. Memory plays a role in health. Holistic health recognizes that we are not separate from the entire web of creation. Therefore any intervention to facilitate the state of health must see the person in relation to all of the parts.

Take Elizabeth, for example. She's an open, loving individual who reports herself to be in a good state of health. She has the energy and the ability to enjoy what is important to her in life; she is active in her church and community and, at the moment, feels at peace with God.

Then she goes for a routine physical examination. The physician finds a breast lump. That piece of information throws Elizabeth out of balance. Her emotions run wild. She can't help thinking of her future and what might happen. Memories of past experiences surface; all that was stable is now unsure.

To intervene holistically requires an understanding of all the parts that make up Elizabeth. She has two small children, she is a wife, she has a career, and she has no family in the local community who can offer support. Her relationship with her church has been mainly giving and caring for others; receiving support from others will not be easy for her. Her mother died of breast cancer, at about this same age. Long-buried grief and anger over her mother's death are suddenly very present.

Elizabeth is more than just a physical body with a breast lump – though that is too often how our medical care systems have treated her. She has relationships, she has roles, she has emotions, memories, and spiritual beliefs. And all of these function within the context of her body

Out of Harmony

If we define health as balance, wholeness, and harmony, then logically illness or disease becomes a lack of balance, lack of harmony, a lack of wholeness. Illness is fragmentation.

Think about when we say, "I am ill," or "I don't feel well." How subtle or obvious do the signs need to be before we pay attention? We are used to breathing in and out with ease and harmony. We expect that our food intake will happen easily and will move through us with ease. We recognize quickly when our breathing or our digestive system is out of balance. Other symptoms may not be as readily noted. Still, our bodies usually call out to us in some manner. Depending on how well we listen, we may catch the signs and symptoms sooner than later. We might not recognize the source of imbalance, but we usually notice the imbalance itself.

I find it helpful to think about life, not as a private entity that we somehow "own," but as a balanced flow of life force moving through us. You can visualize this life force as food, water, or oxygen; or, in my own perceptions, as God's energy flowing through us.

Illness may occur from a physical source. For example, drinking water that is contaminated with harmful bacteria can be an external source of imbalance. Or there may be an emotional source. A constant fear of contaminated water – while camping, perhaps, or while traveling in less-developed countries – can also make one ill. We now know that emotions can open us to illnesses that we could otherwise hold in check. People who have suffered a severe loss, such as a loved one's death or a divorce, are much more likely to come down with anything from colds to cancer and heart attacks during the following 18 months. Or there may be a spiritual source, as in a faith crisis.

Despite the various sources of the illness, the body communicates this imbalance to us. Our job is to learn to listen to the ways our bodies communicate and to value these messages as wisdom.

Where Confusion Reigns

I find a great deal of confusion – to my surprise, especially among church people – about healing.

We need to make a distinction between "healing" and "curing." It's possible to be cured without being healed, and it's equally possible to be healed without being cured. The medical professions, generally, concentrate on cures; it has been cynically said that, in fact, all they seek to cure are the symptoms. If you have blurred sight and an opthalmologist can restore clear vision with prescription eyeglasses, you're considered cured. Healing, however, seeks to repair and restore everything that surrounds the symptom.

Consider, for example, a woman admitted to the hospital for a total hip replacement. She has for many years been unable to walk far. Her disability has isolated her from activities that once gave her life meaning. Her orthopedic surgeon does an excellent job of replacing the hip; the wound heals well; through appropriate physical therapy she is up and walking independently without pain. Contemporary medicine would consider this a cure.

But is she healed? I suggest that she isn't. While in hospital, she enjoyed constant care and attention. There was always someone to talk with, and a chaplain readily available. She finds the thought of going home and being desperately alone again agonizing. Her hip is cured, but her spirit is still broken.

Or consider a hard-driving, hard-drinking, hard-headed business executive. His lifestyle leads to a heart attack. Bypass surgery – or a heart transplant – cures the specific problem. He now has a perfectly sound heart again. But does he have a sound lifestyle? Sound relationships with his staff, his customers? Does he live in better harmony with the world around him?

In such cases, healing would look very different from curing. Growing strong at the broken places means more than physically fixing.

Our word cure comes from the Latin *cura*, meaning care of souls. Today's meaning usually refers only to successful medical treatment, getting rid of or correcting something wrong within the body. Healing, as we use it in this book, comes closer to its original meaning.

Janet Quinn, senior scholar and associate professor at the Center for Human Caring of the Colorado School of Nursing, says that "curing" is a term used in relation to the management of sickness. On the other hand, "healing" refers to the restoration of wholeness. If we measure success by "curing," we will be ultimately 100 percent unsuccessful, because we all die. If we measure success by "healing," we will be 100 percent successful because, even when we die, we live. In *pmc: the Practice of Ministry in Canada*, Quinn wrote,

> The current medical system sees the failure to cure as something to be prevented at any cost – including the cost of the person's humanity. In healing, even death is an opportunity for more healing. Everybody will die. But will everybody die knowing that they are loved? That's the focus of healing.

A Lifelong Challenge

Health or wholeness may first be experienced at a very basic level with our environment; we are fed, warm, and safe. We are then able to explore wholeness within ourselves, a balance within the physiology of our body, our emotions, thoughts and our spirituality.

To examine the wholeness within means to also strive for wholeness with our relationships. This in itself is a lifelong challenge. So as one strives towards healing, one seeks harmony with one's own life, with family, with community, and with the global family that includes all God's creatures. Of prime importance in this journey of healing or restoration of wholeness is the restoration of wholeness and balance with God.

Healing does not occur with a visit to the doctor, or therapist, although that visit may facilitate healing. Nor is healing something done *to* you. Learning to live in harmony, balance and wholeness within the complexity of life is a life-long spiritual journey.

Healing is possible even if the physical body cannot be restored to wholeness. Healing can occur while dying.

I remember my mother's battle with cancer. For many years my mother, Ruby, struggled with cancer. Treatment involved massive doses of radiation as well as surgery. My mother believed that anger she had stored over the years had caused her cancer. She had no proof of this, but without needing proof, she set about healing those old wounds. She had to heal old emotional scars as well as the physical wounds from her surgery and radiation. These were difficult times for her. She had to rally all her resources. But she was a deeply spiritual woman, and her spiritual resources saw her through the toughest times.

At the five-year anniversary of being declared cancer-free, Ruby could claim that she was physically cured. But such a term fails to recognize the transformation that occurred for her – the emotional healing, the spiritual rebirth, much like a phoenix rising from the fire.

After the ten-year anniversary, my mother felt something was again very wrong. Further tests revealed that cancer had recurred in her liver. Within five months, Ruby had died. She died peacefully with her family all around her. So in the end, the cancer was not cured, but I deeply believe that my mother died healed. She absolutely glowed with God's light at the end; she was filled with love; and she was at peace, a source of strength for all of us as we came to terms with "life without Mom."

This is a story about healing from the heart. Although I deeply grieved the loss of my mother, the love present allowed the final healing to happen with grace.

Healing from the Heart

In one of my Healing Touch classes, a student asked, "What are you talking about when you speak of the heart? The heart is simply a physical organ."

Most of us recognize the heart as a physical organ, located in the chest, where it pumps blood to the body. But it is much more than just a pump.

Symbolically, the heart teaches us about service to God. The heart receives revived and refreshed blood from the lungs, and distributes it throughout the body, just as we receive God's grace and gifts generously distributed to all. The heart does not first ask the foot if it has worked hard enough to deserve this gift; it simply gives unconditionally.

The heart also models self-care for us. It receives this enriched blood to nourish and restore itself before it contracts its left ventricle and sends the blood on a journey. Through the venous system, the heart receives blood carrying waste products. The heart does not say, "Not in my back yard!" It doesn't protest that other organs should look after their own wastes. Again unconditionally, it receives this darkened blood and offers it to the lungs, to be restored with new life through another breath.

In our physical bodies the heart is central, and it unifies the whole body through the blood.

In these ways, our bodies teach us about wholeness. All the parts are necessary for the whole to function. Even the darkened blood, the venous blood, teaches us about the symbolism of light and dark in the context of the whole. God is in the whole wonderful process.

Our spiritual ancestors understood these truths intuitively. Most cultures regarded the heart as the seat of emotions, intellect, and will. The heart is cited symbolically throughout the Bible. Both the Hebrew Scriptures and the New Testament described the heart as part of the physical body, but it was also considered the point of contact with God. The heart as the inner point of human personality is open directly to God. It was said to be a place where God knew intimately the thoughts and emotions of the person, and the place where God could transform and Christ could dwell. To take just one example, the Bible says,

> *On the last day of the festival, the great day, while Jesus was*
> *standing there, he cried out, "Let anyone who is thirsty come to*
> *me, and let the one who believes in me drink. As the scripture has*
> *said, 'Out of the believer's heart shall flow rivers of living water.'"*
> (John 7:37-38)

Clearly, he's not speaking literally – rivers do not flow from hearts. What flows from the heart is love, an emotion as necessary for health as water.

We equate love and compassion as expressions of the heart. The highest form of being openhearted is unconditional love. Our hearts remind us to be open to God's love flowing through us, and thus to become channels of divine love.

Our inner life and the divine connect in the heart. Here we begin to live consciously connected to God. True prayer comes from the heart. We understand the qualities of the heart through Paul's famous words:

> *Love is patient; love is kind; love is not envious or boastful or*
> *arrogant or rude. It does not insist on its own way; it is not*
> *irritable or resentful; it does not rejoice in wrongdoing, but rejoices*
> *in the truth. It bears all things, believes all things, hopes all things,*
> *endures all things.* (1 Corinthians 13:4-7)

The physical heart is an expression of this divine love. Divine wisdom keeps it functioning in rhythm with the body's needs, continuously supporting the whole body.

Perhaps it's no coincidence that in a cross-section the physical heart is divided into quadrants – similar in proportion to the Christian cross.

When we speak of healing from the heart, then, we are referring to being instruments of God's healing power. We are connected to the divine, and to the qualities that we refer to as divine. Jesus modeled for us a powerful healing ministry. He modeled love and compassion himself, and he called us to love God with our whole heart and to love one another the same way.

The Heart of God

What does it mean to love another with your whole heart? When we rely on our own energy, we can quickly become drained and burned out. Being present with God's heart means that there are no limits to compassion. Henri Nouwen, the author of more than 30 books who died in 1997, wrote,

> *Every human being has a great yet often unknown gift, to care, to be*
> *compassionate, to become present to the other, to listen, to hear, and*
> *to receive. If the gift would be set free – and made available –*
> *miracles could take place.*

When the compassion and the love of the divine is present with two or more people then all are nourished.

Healing from the heart means to connect to the divine. When we allow the divine to work through us, infinitely more is possible. That's an essential difference between Christian healing and secular healing. We do not act on our own. We do not claim any credit for healings in which we have a part. We are simply conduits through which God's grace can flow to those who need it.

Often when someone is acting as an instrument for God's light and love in facilitating healing, that person is called the "healer." This is not a claim that they are doing the healing; 2 Corinthians 4:7 makes the point:

> *But we have this treasure in clay jars, so that it may be made clear that this extraordinary power belongs to God and does not come from us.*

We are the "clay jars," or, in the words of older translations, "earthen vessels."

That description has a long and honorable history. As Mort Paterson, a United Church minister and Hebrew scholar, explains it, away back in the creation story God formed us "from the dust of the ground" – in Hebrew, *adamah* (the feminine form of *adam*). From this earth, this humus, God made a human, Adam (literally "a being whose life resides in the blood"; the Hebrew *dam* means "blood"). Then God breathed into Adam's nostrils "the breath of life."

Our origins in clay remind us that we are creatures of the earth, blessed by the breath or Spirit of God.

So healing has three components: the healer, the person seeking healing, and God. Individuals who engage in the practice of healing are instruments; we learn and practice necessary skills. But the power and potential for healing always comes from God. The person asking for the healing is also actively involved. Morton Kelsey in his book *Healing and Christianity* describes it this way:

> *When I truly love another human being, and the other is open to that love, the divine communes within itself, using two human beings as instruments.*

The Skills of Healing

That's an awesome responsibility. It's not one we can simply assume for ourselves. Wayne began piano lessons at four years of age, before his hands had much of a reach. His physical body needed to grow. But so did other sides of him. After 16 years of lessons, he was attempting Franz Liszt's Hungarian Rhapsody no. 2. But after listening to Wayne, his teacher said, "Put it away. You haven't lived long enough to play that one yet."

In healing as in piano playing, there are skills to develop. They may take time and experience. Even the saints engaged in many hours of prayer and meditation daily to connect with and become divine channels. The physical body, nervous system, and brain all require consistent training. Only then can they properly transmit the power, the energy, the grace, love, compassion and other divine qualities required to facilitate healing that flow from God. Florence Nightingale, known as the founder of modern nursing, called this practice to connect with the divine, "growth in grace."

The path of an individual committed to being a vessel for God's healing power is an evolutionary one. It requires commitment, spiritual practice, and dedication to self-growth. The human may be called a healer, but it is always God who heals.

Healing comes from God. We are merely the instruments,
flesh and blood born of the earth, who carry God's healing to those who need it.
*But if we fail to perform that function, says **Flora Litt**,*
we are betraying our heritage, our tradition, and our faith.

2

The Biblical Basis
for Christian Healing

The Hebrew Scriptures, often called the Old Testament, contain a number of healing stories. They are apparently there for a variety of purposes. Some demonstrate God's power on Israel's behalf; some respond to prayers entreating God to heal individuals. Taken together, these stories give evidence that those whom God anointed, long before the coming of Jesus (God's anointed One), were also vessels and channels of God's power.

One of the first healing stories appears in Exodus 4:6-8. God makes Moses' hand leprous and then restores it. This was a sign to the people that Moses was God's chosen servant, the one to whom God spoke, the one through whom God's power was worked.

The wonderful story of Elisha raising the Shunammite woman's son is told in 2 Kings 4:8-37. The child has died. His mother brings Elisha to the boy's room. Elisha lays his body over the child and the child revives. In answer to prayer, the mighty power of God moved through God's chosen prophet.

In the next chapter, 2 Kings 5:1-19, Elisha instructs Naaman in what he must do to heal his leprosy. In this familiar story, when Naaman finally does obey Elisha and wash seven times in the Jordan, he is completely healed.

Elisha must have been viewed as a very powerful healer indeed. Following the death and burial of Elisha, this incident takes place:

As a man was being buried, a marauding band was seen and the
man was thrown into the grave of Elisha; as soon as the man
touched the bones of Elisha, he came to life and stood on his feet.
(2 Kings 13:21)

The energy of God remained as a healing force, even in Elisha's bones!

All these incidents show how the power of the almighty God could act through chosen individuals. But there are also instances where God responded directly to individuals. 2 Kings 20:1-7 tells of Hezekiah who "became sick and was at the point of death." The prophet Isaiah had announced that Hezekiah would die. But because of Hezekiah's bitter tears, pleading, and praying, God's decision was reversed. God spoke again through Isaiah, saying,

I have heard your prayer, I have seen your tears;
indeed I will heal you... (2 Kings 20:5)

Other references are,
1 Kings 13:4-6   Jeroboam's hand, withered and restored
2 Kings 6:8-23   Blinded eyes opened

The Healing Ministry of Jesus

The New Testament story of salvation begins with the familiar words in the message of the angel at the time of Jesus' birth:

To you is born this day in the city of David a Savior, who is the
Messiah, the Lord. (Luke 2:11)

The Greek word soter (savior) was used to refer to philosophers, statesmen, and physicians. Its use suggested salvation from meaningless life, from crises of a social and political nature – and from disease. The New Testament uses this word uniquely for Jesus of Nazareth. As Savior, Jesus came with a mission: delivering people from sin and sickness, and bringing new meaning into their lives.

Jesus announced his saving mission, declaring himself to be the promised Messiah, the one sent and empowered to fulfill the prophecy of Isaiah. There were other understandings of a Savior, of course. Most of these took David, the conquering king, as their model. But Isaiah had an inspired vision of "the suffering servant," one whose life epitomized compassion, loyalty, and self-sacrifice.

Jesus took Isaiah's model for his ministry. It spoke to God's continuing purpose to make people whole, to meet every dimension of human need.

In the synagogue in his home town of Nazareth, Jesus read from Isaiah, in his Hebrew Scriptures:

> *The Spirit of the Lord is upon me, because he has anointed me to*
> *bring good news to the poor. He has sent me to proclaim release to*
> *the captives and recovery of sight to the blind, to let the oppressed*
> *go free, to proclaim the year of the Lord's favor.* (Luke 4:18-19)

Later in Jesus' ministry, John the Baptist, imprisoned by King Herod, sent his disciples – Jesus was not the only person who had followers! – to find out if Jesus really was the long-promised Messiah. In Luke 7:19b, 21-22, they asked,

> *"Are you the one who is to come, or are we to wait for another?"*
> *Jesus had just then cured many people of diseases, plagues,*
> *and evil spirits, and had given sight to many who were blind.*
> *And he answered them [John's disciples] saying, "Go and*
> *tell John what you have seen and heard: the blind receive their sight,*
> *the lame walk, the lepers are cleansed, the deaf hear, the dead*
> *are raised, the poor have good news brought to them."*

The number of texts that link Jesus' ministry to healing are overwhelming.

God's Healing Agent

In Chapter 1, Rochelle makes the point that healers do not heal out of their own power. That corresponds to Jesus' own assertions that he could do nothing on his own, but that all he did was a revelation of the works of his Father, even to the raising of the dead.

> *Jesus said to them, "Very truly, I tell you, the Son can do nothing*
> *on his own, but only what he sees the Father doing; for*
> *whatever the Father does, the Son does likewise. The Father*
> *loves the Son and shows him all that he himself is doing;*
> *and he will show him greater works than these, so that you*
> *will be astonished. Indeed just as the Father raises the dead and*
> *gives them life, so also the Son gives life to whomever he wishes."*
> (John 5:19-21)

Matthew records that the healings of Jesus were recognized by the crowds to be the work of the Covenant God of Israel.

> *Jesus... passed along the Sea of Galilee, and he went up the*
> *mountain, where he sat down. Great crowds came to him,*
> *bringing with them the lame, the maimed, the blind, the mute,*
> *and many others. They put them at his feet, and he cured them, so*
> *that the crowd was amazed... And they praised the God of Israel.*
> (Matthew 15: 29b-31)

We need never wonder whether God *wants* to heal. To make people whole was and is always God's intention and will. It was evidenced in the Hebrew Scriptures, predicted by the prophets, and demonstrated by Jesus. We need only look at what Jesus did. As he said,

> *Whoever has seen me has seen the Father.* (John 14:9b)

When a leper came to Jesus, he threw himself down before Jesus and begged,

> *"If you want to, Lord, you can make me clean." Jesus stretched out*
> *his hand, placed it on the leper, saying, "Certainly I want to.*
> *Be clean!"* (Luke 5:12b-13, J.B. Phillips paraphrase)

Jesus preached this fundamental message and confirmed it with signs and wonders: the reign of God is at hand; salvation has come to God's people. The crowds were astonished; they declared among themselves that he must be the Messiah.

About one-quarter of the gospels are concerned with healings in Jesus' ministry. They record 26 individual healing miracles and 14 healings of larger numbers of people. This is apart from the power delegated by Jesus to his disciples to heal under his authority.

There is, in fact, more record of the healing ministry in the gospels than of any other topic or experience. Jesus entered into every segment of society, into the lives of needy people wherever he encountered them. All who came to Jesus for healing were healed. He made no distinctions, turned no one away, and found no case beyond his power to heal. And John tells us (in John 20:30) that the works of Jesus recorded in his gospel were only a few of those Jesus performed!

Now Jesus did many other signs in the presence of his disciples,
which are not written in this book.

A List of Jesus' Miracles of Healing

(A miracle may be understood to be any event in which one sees a revelation of God.)

	Matthew	Mark	Luke	John
Miracles of healing illness				
Man with leprosy	8:2-4	1:40-42	5:12-13	
Centurion's servant	8:5-13		7:1-10	
Peter's mother-in-law	8:14-15	1:30-31	4:38-39	
Two Gadarene demoniacs	8:28-34	5:1-15	8:27-35	
Paralyzed man	9:2-7	2:3-12	5:18-25	
Woman with hemorrhages	9:20-22	5:25-29	8:43-48	
Two blind men	9:27-31			
Mute/demon-possessed man	9:32-33			
Man with a withered hand	12:10-13	3:1-5	6:6-10	
Blind/mute/demon-possession	12:22		11:14	
Canaanite woman's daughter	15:21-28	7:24-30		
Boy with a demon	17:14-18	9:17-29	9:38-42	
Two blind men (including Bartimaeus)	20:29-34	10:46-52	18:35-43	
Deaf man with speech impediment		7:31-37		
Possessed man in synagogue		1:23-26	4:33-35	
Blind man at Bethsaida		8:22-25		
Crippled woman			13:11-13	
Man with dropsy			14:1-4	
Ten men with leprosy			17:11-19	
The high priest's slave			22:50-51	
Official's son at Capernaum				4:46-54
Sick man at pool of Beth-zatha				5:1-9
Man born blind				9:1-7
Miracles of raising the dead				
Jairus' daughter	9:18-25	5:22-42	8:41-56	
Widow's son at Nain			7:11-15	
Lazarus				11:1-44

The Ministry of Jesus' Followers

Jesus expected his followers to share in his healing ministry. The references are again overwhelming, both in the gospels and in the story of the fledgling church of the first century.

> *Jesus summoned his twelve disciples and gave them authority over unclean spirits, to cast them out, and to cure every disease and every sickness.* (Matthew 10:1)

He sent them out "to the lost sheep of Israel" with the same ministry as his own, commanding them to

> *proclaim the good news, "The kingdom of heaven has come near. Cure the sick, raise the dead, cleanse lepers, cast out demons."*
> (Matthew 10:7-8a)

And this they did as they

> *went through the villages, bringing the good news and curing diseases everywhere.* (Luke 9:6)

And again Jesus

> *appointed seventy others and sent them on ahead of him in pairs to every town and place where he himself intended to go.*
> (Luke 10:1)

They returned with joyous news, reporting,

> *Lord, in your name even the demons submit to us.* (Luke 10:17b)

The disciples were not always successful. But Jesus left his disciples with no doubt that they were to continue his healing ministry. In fact he amazingly promised they would do even more. They would ask anything in his name and he would do it, interceding with God on their behalf:

The one who believes in me will also do the works that I do and, in fact, will do greater works than these, because I am going to the Father. I will do whatever you ask in my name, so that the Father may be glorified in the Son. If in my name you ask me for anything, I will do it. (John 14:12-14)

The fulfillment of his promise began with the pouring out of the Spirit on the day of Pentecost. Immediately the same healing power that Jesus had exhibited in his life and ministry began to be manifested. Acts 2:43 relates,

Awe came upon everyone, because many wonders and signs were being done by the apostles.

Peter and John were so emboldened that they risked healing a crippled beggar by the gate to the temple, right on the doorsteps of the authorities who conspired to crucify Jesus. Peter made it very clear to the people that what they (the apostles) did was in the name of Jesus of Nazareth (Acts 3:1-10). The power of God, through Christ, enabled these miracles so that the people might believe the message the apostles spoke. The glory, if any, belonged to God.

What Jesus had done when he was alive, his disciples continued to do after his death. The parallels are striking: healing the lame, the sick, the paralyzed… Acts 5:15-16 tells us how great was the power of Christ that moved through the apostles to heal.

They even carried out the sick into the streets, and laid them on cots and mats, in order that Peter's shadow might fall on some of them as he came by. A great number of people would also gather…bringing the sick and those tormented by unclean spirits, and they were all cured.

Healing marked the ministry of all the apostles, not just in those days immediately after Pentecost. (See Acts 14:3, 8-10; 16:16-18; 19:11-12; 20:9-12 and 28:8-9.) The healing ministry of Philip is recorded in Acts 8:5-8; in chapter 9:17-19 a disciple named Ananias is used by God to restore the sight of Saul after his conversion and blindness on the road to Damascus.

It's interesting to examine the kinds of healing that took place, and the ways they were accomplished.

Firstly, we see that healing applied to everything from apparently slight ailments to severe ones, even to death. The spectrum included

1. Relatively minor discomfort, like that of Peter's mother-in-law's fever (Matthew 8:14-15).
2. Advanced stages of disease, as in the "man covered with leprosy" (Luke 5:12-13).
3. Congenital conditions, like the men blind from birth (John 9:1-12) and crippled from birth (Acts 3:1-10).
4. Chronic conditions, like the "woman who had been suffering with hemorrhages twelve years" (Matthew 9:20-22), and the man by the pool of Bethsaida "who had been ill for 38 years" (John 5:5-9).
5. Terminal conditions, those at the point of death like the royal official's son (John 4:46b-53), and Jairus' daughter (Mark 5:21-23, 35-42), and Lazarus who was not only dead but already buried (John 11:38-44).

Secondly, the causes of physical distress included

1. Illness as a result of accident, as when a snoozing Eutychus fell out the window (!) while Paul was preaching (Acts 20:9-12).
2. Wounding by attack, like the ear of the slave of the High Priest severed by Peter's sword during Jesus' arrest (Luke 22:50-51).
3. Distress of mind and heart, as in the case of the paralytic (Matthew 9:2-7).
4. Demonic oppression, as with the Canaanite woman's daughter "tormented by a demon" (Matthew 15:22-28), or demonic possession (Matthew 17:14-18).

Thirdly, although Jesus usually healed in the presence of those in need, and most often by some form of physical touch, there were also occasions when he healed at a distance:

1. Roman centurion's servant (Matthew 8:5-13)
2. Two Gadarene demoniacs (Mark 5:1-20)
3. Canaanite woman's daughter (Mark 7:24-30)
4. Official's son at Capernaum (John 4:46-53)

Healing Never Became Routine

In all of these examples, there was no standard healing method. Although human suffering and a cry for help always evoked compassion in Jesus, his way of healing was unique to each individual's need. He touched; he spoke; he listened. He restored to community. And he often employed various methods in combination.

Jesus had an inner knowing, a spiritual gift of discernment, that helped him respond to each situation. Luke, in telling how the Pharisees watched Jesus to see if he would cure on the Sabbath, says,

> *Even though he knew what they were thinking, he said to the man*
> *who had the withered hand, "Come and stand here."* (Luke 6:8)

Jesus had an amazingly penetrating way of knowing facts about people. He knew the man he healed on the Sabbath by the pool of Beth-zatha *"had been there a long time"* (John 5:6). He knew the personal history of the woman at the well in Samaria: *"You have had five husbands, and the one you have now is not your husband"* (John 4:18a).

He saw through outward behavior. So he berated the scribes for their double standard:

> *For you are like whitewashed tombs, which on the outside look*
> *beautiful, but inside they are full of the bones of the dead and of*
> *all kinds of filth.* (Matthew 23:27)

For such persons as these, Jesus knew that only repentance and a change of heart could allow healing for their souls.

Since he perceived the heart, mind and spirit of a person, discerning their inner condition, he knew the healing method required to restore each one.

1. Touch

The practice of laying on hands goes back long before Jesus. Leviticus 16:21-22 says that Moses' brother Aaron laid both his hands on the head of a live goat and confessed the sins of the people, healing the people of their guilt and transferring their sins to the goat who would bear them off into the wilderness. (From this origin, we get the term "scapegoat.") With a different purpose, Moses laid his hands on Joshua to commission him as Moses' successor (Numbers 27:18, 22-23).

While there are few accounts in the Hebrew Scriptures of healing through the laying on of hands, other healings did depend on physical contact. When Elijah restored the widow's son to life,

> *he stretched himself upon the child three times, and cried out to*
> *the Lord, "O Lord, my God, let this child's life come into him*
> *again."* (1 Kings 17:21)

Similarly, when Elisha raised the Shunammite's son, 2 Kings 4:32-37 says,

> *When Elisha came into the house, he saw the child lying dead on*
> *his bed. So he…got up on the bed and lay upon the child, putting*
> *his mouth upon his mouth, his eyes upon his eyes, and his hand*
> *upon his hands; and while he lay bent over him, the flesh of the*
> *child became warm. …The child sneezed seven times, and the*
> *child opened his eyes.*

These two passages are fascinating. Somehow, the energy fields of the two were so united that each child's body became enlivened by the strong energy of God flowing through the prophet.

Jesus continued that tradition. He frequently touched others. He blessed children, washed feet, healed injuries or illness, and raised people from death. His touch embodied the acceptance, caring, and love of God. His willingness to touch modeled his servanthood and his awareness that the wisdom and power of God flowed through him.

Jesus also allowed himself to be touched, washed, embraced, anointed. To allow or invite others to touch him was an act of openness and acceptance.

Most of Jesus' healings involved touch. This in itself was heretical and revolutionary, for he lived in a society of touching taboos. Social and religious rules rigorously defined what one could and could not touch. If one touched something or someone considered unclean, one became unclean oneself. A leper was among the most unclean, as was a dead body. A menstruating woman was also considered unclean. Contact with any of these required following elaborate rituals of purification before one was once more acceptable to the community.

Jesus broke all these taboos. He touched lepers and dead bodies. He responded to the touch of a menstruating woman. Regardless of how the community labeled a person, he freely reached out to touch in love. His authority came from God, and he was not bound by human regulations. But while his response of compassion was most often immediate, his way of touching varied, because he discerned the best way for healing the root of any dis-ease.

He touched the children (Matthew 19:13-15), not only to bless them, but that the disciples might clearly understand the inestimable worth of every person in God's sight. His touch became a parable of the importance of coming before God with the openness and receptivity of a childlike heart. He touched blind eyes (Matthew 9:29; 20:34), put his fingers in deaf ears, and touched a mute tongue (Mark 7:33). He touched a hand to disperse a fever (Matthew 8:15). And he laid hands on great numbers of people:

> *...all those who had any who were sick with various kinds of diseases brought them to him; and he laid his hands on each of them and cured them.* (Luke 4:40)

He touched his disciples in the washing of their feet. It was an act normally reserved for a servant – or, if there were no servant available, of a woman or child. The disciples were shocked. But he did it because they needed to be cured of pride! He became their servant to teach them servanthood and humility.

> *If I, your Lord and Teacher, have washed your feet, you also ought to wash one another's feet. For I have set you an example...* (John 13:14-15)

People reached out to touch Jesus themselves, for they felt the healing energy radiating from him. Luke records,

> *And all in the crowd were trying to touch him, for power came out from him and healed all of them.* (Luke 6:19)

Jesus felt the touch of the woman with the hemorrhage in Luke 8:44-46. And in Mark 6:56, we read how people begged that the sick

> *might touch even the fringe of his cloak; and all who touched it were healed.*

The disciples, too, used touch in their ministry. In Acts 3:7, Peter took the crippled beggar *"by the right hand and raised him up."* As well, people reached out to them as they passed by, desiring that even Peter's shadow might touch the sick and heal them (Acts 5:15).

Yet clearly this was not a power to be taken lightly. In Acts 8:4-25 we read the story of a man named Simon, newly baptized by Philip. When he saw Peter and John lay hands on people to receive the Holy Spirit, he affronted the disciples by attempting to bribe them. He said,

"Give me also this power so that anyone on whom I lay my hands
may receive the Holy Spirit." But Peter said to him, "May your
silver perish with you, because you thought you could obtain
God's gift with money! You have no part or share in this, for your
heart is not right before God. Repent therefore of this wickedness
of yours, and pray to the Lord that, if possible, the intent of your
heart may be forgiven you." (Acts 8:19-22)

2. Spoken word

But Jesus did more than just touch. As an expression of his love, he also spoke with people, and listened to them.

His Hebrew culture had long recognized the power of the word – especially the word of God. The Christian tradition adds something new. The word that God sent out to heal became the Word-made-flesh (John 1:1), a human being – Jesus the Christ. And when Jesus spoke, this same power manifested through him.

Sometimes Jesus first spoke forgiveness, or commended faith, or taught, before a physical healing. Words were necessary, either to break down blocks or build up trust. Often he commanded healing or rebuked the sickness directly. He expressed authority through the spoken word. To the leper in Matthew 8:3, Jesus said, *"Be made clean!" "Be opened!"* he ordered the ears of the deaf man in Mark 7:34. *"Go!"* he said to the demons in Matthew 8:32.

He also used words to instruct people what to do after their healing. The blind man was to go and wash in the pool of Siloam.

Then he went and washed and came back able to see. (John 9:7)

The paralytic was commanded to pick up his bed and walk.

And he stood up and went to his home. (Matthew 9:7)

The lepers were required to show themselves to the priest.

And as they went they were made clean. (Luke 17:14b)

Jesus' healing through spoken word also extended to his conversations with people, his teaching, and preaching. His words and deeds were not separate. Together they served his mission of healing people's relationship to God and one another. Through his words, he addressed the physical, emotional, mental, spiritual or social dis-ease of persons:

- The rich ruler (Luke 18:18-30)
- Jesus and Zacchaeus (Luke 19:1-10)
- The woman of Samaria at Jacob's well (John 4:1-42)
- The woman caught in adultery (John 8:2-11)

3. Prayer and Fasting

Jesus also depended on what we would call "spiritual discipline." He told the disciples that deliverance ministry, healing by exorcism, could only be done by prayer (Mark 9:29).

The scriptures do not actually refer to Jesus' fasting from food, other than during his time of temptation in the wilderness. Indeed, he was directly criticized for eating and drinking, almost too readily. His critics called him "a glutton and a drunkard" (Matthew 11:19). But since fasting was a Jewish custom, it may well have been part of his practice.

As we read in the Sermon on the Mount, Jesus was not opposed to fasting, just to a self-righteous and public display of it. So he said,

> *When you fast, put oil on your head and wash your face, so that*
> *your fasting may be seen not by others but by your Father who is*
> *in secret; and your Father who sees in secret will reward you.*
> (Matthew 6:17-18)

We do know that as well as his regular prayer in temple and synagogue, he often fasted from people! He needed to get away from the crowds from time to time, for rest and renewal. Though the power that came through him to heal was from God, he was a human vehicle, and as such he must have felt the effect of constantly being a channel of such power.

> *He made his disciples get into the boat and go on ahead to the*
> *other side, to Bethsaida, while he dismissed the crowd. After*
> *saying farewell to them, he went up on the mountain to pray.*
> (Mark 6:45-46)

He spent long nights alone in prayer and meditation, or arose early to go off by himself.

*In the morning, while it was still very dark, he got up and went
out to a deserted place, and there he prayed.* (Mark 1:35)

Through prayer, Jesus kept himself prepared, attuned, and built up in the Spirit.
From his close communion with God, he received guidance and gathered the
strength he needed for teaching, preaching, and healing. Through this openness, the flow of the healing power was kept clear and strong.

4. Substances

We don't know if Jesus ever used oil in his healings. But his disciples certainly did. When Jesus sent out the twelve,

*They cast out many demons, and anointed with oil many who
were sick and cured them.* (Mark 6:13)

After Jesus' death, the disciples continued to anoint, and they taught the church
to use anointing in healing of the sick (James 5:14).

But Jesus did not hesitate to use other substances to promote healing. Jesus
anointed with saliva and mud in healing the blind man in John 9:6. Whatever
he touched was infused with power to heal. Even the robe Jesus wore radiated
a powerful spiritual energy. The disciples had been present when healings resulted from Jesus' clothing being touched.

This also happened to Paul, later.

*God did extraordinary miracles through Paul, so that when the
handkerchiefs or aprons that had touched his skin were brought to the
sick, their diseases left them, and the evil spirits came out of them.*
(Acts 19:11-12)

Anointing in the East was a common practice:
- As a mark of respect (Luke 7:46)
- For burial (Mark 14:8;16:1)
- Sacred action for anointing prophets (1 Kings 19:16), for anointing priests
  (Exodus 28:41), and for anointing kings (1 Samuel 9:16)
- As treatment for the sick and wounded (Isaiah 1:6; Luke 10:34)
  In its sacred use, oil symbolizes the presence and action of the Holy Spirit
  in both the Hebrew Scriptures and the New Testament. God instructed
  Moses how the oil for anointing should be made, and for what purposes:

This shall be my holy anointing oil throughout your generations.
It shall not be used in any ordinary anointing of the body, and
you shall make no other like it in composition; it is holy, and it
shall be holy to you. (Exodus 30:31-32)

The holy anointing oil, unlike any other oil in scripture, symbolized the cleansing, consecration, and active presence of God's Holy Spirit.

The words "Messiah" (Hebrew) and "Christ" (Greek) both mean "the Anointed One." Jesus the Christ came as the One anointed by God in fulfillment of the prophecies, the One who would save God's people. The elders who were to anoint with oil when praying for the sick were among those who themselves had received the divine anointing of Pentecost, the Holy Spirit (James 5:14). And God has anointed us through Christ with the same Spirit.

So the apostle John writes to the believers:

As for you, the anointing that you received from him abides in
you, and so you do not need anyone to teach you. But as his
anointing teaches you about all things, and is true and is not a
lie...abide in him. (1 John 2:27)

Christians of early centuries commonly prayed for healing for their relatives and friends, using oil blessed by the bishop and distributed by the church for anointing the sick. As in the days of Jesus, the effectiveness of this practice built faith and won converts. Gregory of Nyssa, who lived around 335-395 CE wrote, "Healing is the main door through which people come to a knowledge of the truth."

Healing Spreads Like Ripples

The call to set captives free, to liberate the oppressed, to minister to the poor, and to heal the sick is still Christ's mission and ours. Our mandate as individual disciples and as the church is the same as that given to the seventy Jesus sent out – to proclaim the reign of God and to heal (Luke 9:2). As disciples and *"ambassadors for Christ"* (2 Corinthians 5:20a), we do this through promoting peace and justice, and by performing acts of mercy, including healing.

Clearly, in the early church, healing was not expected to be limited to the apostles. In writing to the Corinthians, Paul mentions gifts of healing among other gifts of the Spirit given to the church. Paul's listing of spiritual gifts implies that some persons may have given special attention to healing as a calling, but the gift of healing was never considered to be owned by any particular group. It was, and is, given to the whole community of faith. James, the pastor and leader of the Jerusalem church, addressed the Christian church in general when he wrote,

> *Are any among you sick? They should call for the elders of the*
> *church and have them pray over them, anointing them with oil in*
> *the name of the Lord. The prayer of faith will save the sick, and*
> *the Lord will raise them up; and anyone who has committed sins*
> *will be forgiven. Therefore confess your sins to one another, and*
> *pray for one another, so that you may be healed. The prayer of the*
> *righteous is powerful and effective.* (James 5:14-16)

James obviously assumed that the church elders would be prepared to do this!

In the first chapters of his book, James describes sins that create *"disputes and conflicts"* and destroy relationships. He appears to relate disharmony in the community to ensuing suffering and sickness. More than 19 centuries ago, he understood intuitively the connection between spiritual and relational disorder and the physical illness. He recognizes confession and forgiveness as essential for clearing blocks to healing.

*Healing is an ancient and honorable practice. Whether by the laying on of hands, anointing with oil, or any other method, all civilizations have practiced healing in one way or another. In our time, **Flora Litt** finds heartening the new mood in which a variety of disciplines learn from and respect one another.*

3

From the Old to the New

Healing of the sick through laying on of hands, praying, and anointing with various substances has been known from the earliest days of the human race. We can trace the practice as far back in history as we are able to go, and it may well have been prevalent before the days of written history. It is practiced among all races today. It seems to arise from an instinctive awareness in the human mind that healing is intimately connected with touch. Ancient Indians, Egyptians, Jews, and Chinese were all familiar with this form of healing. Ancient rock carvings in Egypt show healers treating patients with one hand on the stomach and the other on the back – postures and positions sometimes startlingly similar to today's. Early explorers reported similar practices in China.

The Egyptians learned from the ancient Yogi teachers and then established their own schools of healing. The Hebrews and Assyrians are also believed to have obtained much of their knowledge through Egyptian channels.

The Greeks obtained their knowledge of healing from Egypt and India. Early Greek physicians performed their healing principally through laying on of hands and manipulating affected parts of the body. This work belonged to the priesthood. The temples of Aesculapius, devoted to the cure of disease, were the hospitals of the ancient Greek world. The priests healed by breathing on the diseased parts of the body and by stroking with the hands.

To the general public the healing process was a mystery. Hippocrates, considered the founder of modern medicine – physicians still adhere to the Hippocratic Oath – wrote, "The affections suffered by the body, the soul sees quite well with shut eyes."

Early Christianity expected that physical cures would accompany the laying on of hands in baptism, communion, and special services for the sick. They celebrated cures of various ailments as evidence of God's presence in Christ among them.

For those early Christians, whose living conditions were as severe as in any developing country today, sickness represented the ever-present threat of death. In that context, healing touch functioned as much to encourage faith in Christ's victory over death, and hope in his imminent return, as to channel healing energies for specific ills. As a result of healing touch, the first Christians expected not just healing for the body, but a deeper wholeness: strength, forgiveness of sins, new life, and protection of body, mind, and spirit. So from the beginning, healing touch was not essentially a private moment but was shaped by the church's efforts to encourage wholeness and community in the harsh realities of life.

Ancient Druid priests in Ireland and elsewhere also performed cures by breathing on diseased parts and stroking with the hands as part of their religious ceremonies and rites. It has been reported that St. Patrick healed the blind in Ireland by placing his hands upon their eyes. St. Bernard is said to have cured 11 blind people and enabled 18 lame persons to regain the use of their limbs, all in one day. And in Cologne, Germany, he is said to have cured 12 lame people, 3 dumb persons, and 10 deaf ones by laying on of hands.

During the first eight centuries after Christ, church members experienced healing touch in the sacraments and in their homes. The laying on of hands, along with anointing with oil, was performed by families as needed. United Church of Canada minister Chris McMullen, in his 1995 research paper on *The Ministry of Prayer for Healing*, notes,

> *The Venerable Bede (d. 735) meticulously records acts of both*
> *conventional and miraculous healing, always associated with the*
> *laying on of hands and/or anointing and prayer, in the early*
> *Celtic churches of Britain. This does not seem to have become an*
> *exclusive ordinance for clergy until the ninth century. Peter*
> *Lombard seems to have been the first to identify the ritual as one*
> *of the Seven Sacraments, restricting such to a clerical act, as*
> *opposed to a prayer resource available to all Christians.*

Care for the Soul Rather than the Body

St. Jerome said, "Plato located the soul of man in the head; Christ located it in the heart."

All through the second and third centuries, the Christian community practiced and taught healing. Most writers of this time attest to healings, often leading to conversion.

But early in the second century, the philosophy of Plato underwent a revival. It would affect the healing ministry of the early church. For although the writers of the Bible saw a person as an integrated whole – spirit, soul and body – the philosophy of the Neoplatonists saw spirit and body as separate. They taught that a person had a higher nature consisting of soul, intellect, and will; and a lower nature of body, emotions, and appetites.

Eventually, the church began to be influenced by the secular thought of the time. No longer did it minister to the whole person, but only to the spirit.

In popular thinking, the power of healing gradually passed from the people themselves, to priests, to monarchs. History reports that Pyrrhus, the king of Epirus, had the power of curing colic and diseases of the spleen by touching the persons affected, and Emperor Vespasian reportedly cured nervous diseases, lameness, blindness and other infirmities through the laying on of hands. The Roman historian Pliny chronicles that in ancient days, some men were able to cure serpent bites with their touch. Emperor Hadrian applied the points of his fingers to people who had dropsical diseases, and King Olaf also effected instantaneous healings by laying his hands on the sufferer. Early kings in England and in France healed goiter and throat troubles with what was called the "King's touch." And the Counts of Hapsburg were said to be able to cure stammering with a kiss.

In 313 CE, Emperor Constantine made Christianity the official religion of the Roman empire. As worship became more structured, the exercise of charismatic gifts including healing declined. Augustine explained this reversal by teaching that the supernatural gifts had been for the establishing of the church and were now no longer needed. Paradoxically, as if in correction of his error, in Augustine's own declining years the Spirit moved in his community with many remarkable healing miracles being done!

In the centuries following, the church continued to care for the sick. Monasteries were centers of medical care and learning during the Middle Ages. The monks were instructed that since medicine had been created by God, and since it is God who gives health and restores life, they should turn to God, the Creator, for healing.

But in 1123, the Catholic Church's Lateran Council issued an edict that forbade the clergy to care for the sick – except as spiritual directors. Plato's philosophy had taken over the church: the soul was important, and the body with its evil inclinations was to be brought under submission.

By the 13th century the practice of prayer and anointing with oil for healing had become last rites for the dying. This act was meant to ensure the soul's eternal salvation rather than provide healing for the whole person.

During the Protestant Reformation, Calvin and Luther maintained this concern for the soul rather than the body. They did not support charismatic gifts of healing, but rather the use of "ordinary prayer" in caring for the sick.

A Sign of Power and Authority

Through the Middle Ages, both church and culture grew preoccupied with levels of authority, the very thing Jesus warned against in Matthew 20:25-28. In this period, healing touch disappeared among the laity. It became what Zach Thomas in *Healing Touch* calls "power touch," exercised only by religious and political authorities.

Later, with the birth of science in the 16th and 17th centuries, scientists were so enamored of the powers of the mind that they had little regard for the body. Both "healing touch" and "power touch" were considered superstitions of the past; "no touch" became the accepted scientific philosophy. Eventually, the "no touch" philosophy in the helping professions, religious communities, and families had an adverse effect, in some cases resulting in abusive touch – what Thomas called "touch gone wrong."

There were exceptions to this progressive decline of interest in healing body as well as soul. In the 18th century, John Wesley not only prayed for healing, he also experimented with a healing apparatus. While living and working in London, stirred by concern for so many supposed incurables, he made use of this invention, a direct-current voltage generator. In his journal, he records various occasions when he "electrified people." He claimed that he had helped hundreds, even thousands.

Still, by the beginning of the 20th century, no major Christian church had a theology of prayer for the healing intervention of God through gifts of the Spirit.

The mainline church has for the most part limited laying on of hands to baptism, confirmation, and ordination. It has not been associated with healing – though healing has continued to happen through participation in the Eucharist, counseling, etc. But the work Jesus commissioned us to carry out, and which our bodies naturally enjoy, calls for touching that facilitates the healing process.

The Recovery of Healing Ministries

In spite of this trend, the church's healing ministry never did disappear entirely. Apart from revival and crusade-type gatherings, some independent, and usually charismatic ministries continued to offer prayer for healing of the whole person.

In our own century there have been a number of authentic "faith healers" – Agnes Sanford, Kathryn Kuhlman, and Olga and Ambrose Worrall had outstanding healing gifts. And, of course, there were others who were not authentic.

Today the blessing of loving, healing touch is being reclaimed in the church once more as the Spirit guides the unfolding of the ministry of prayer for healing in the name of Jesus. The wisdom of the Hebrew understanding is again respected, and the church is learning intentionally and actively to care for the whole person once more.

Starting in 1962, Vatican II revolutionized the Roman Catholic practice of healing. Today the Rite of Anointing is once again prayer for wholeness in life rather than preparation for death. The Anglican Church of Canada has long had a healing liturgy, and its Order of St. Luke has contributed significantly to the revival of healing in the church. In recent years other mainline denominations have made liturgies of prayer for healing available to clergy, and encouraged again the participation of lay people in anointing and laying on of hands in healing prayer services. In Great Britain, church-supported residential healing centers have come into being, such as Burrswood, Crowshurst, and Green Pastures. In these centers persons are treated holistically; physicians attend to physical conditions and counselors and clergy attend to soul and spirit.

Healing Ministries Resurface

The rediscovery of the ministry of healing has come at the right time. Life on our planet has fallen out of its primal balance. Woods have been raped; seas and skies have lost their pristine cleanliness. Pavement does not breathe as do meadows and trees, nor do oiled waters support life as clear lakes and mountain streams do. Our planet needs healing. And we, the inhabitants of this planet, need healing.

As a global society we suffer relationally, and need healing as a human race. Who among us is in perfect health, physically, emotionally, mentally, and spiritually all the days of our life? To be human is to recognize that we are part of the imbalance, as both contributor and victim.

The need for healing in the human being may appear initially as dis-ease at a spiritual, emotional, mental, physical or relational level. But the whole person is affected, no matter where the need initially appears. Today we openly acknowledge that much physical illness begins at non-physical levels – some would say all illness does. While a few may yet believe that our physical, mental, emotional and spiritual aspects exist in separate compartments, religion, medicine, and science all affirm this is not so.

It has been said that the body is "spirit incognito." There is spirit in every cell, supporting the life and activity of every cell. The "spiritual" is not separate from the rest of being, but rather interpenetrates the whole.

While specialists prescribe for the physical, and therapists for the psychological, the contribution of the spiritual counselor to the individual's belief system and spiritual practices is invaluable in restoring balance and harmony. Knowing this, 12-Step and Alcoholics Anonymous Programs include a spiritual component. Many therapists today may refer a client to a pastor or spiritual director to assist in exploring their innate spirituality or to deal with a faith or forgiveness concern.

Complementary Practices Flourish

Increasingly, people are unwilling to hand over full responsibility for their healing to medical practitioners. Many want to be involved in their own healing process, which can include anything from hands on or off the body treatments, homeopathy, vitamin therapy, nutrition, yoga, or prayer. Credible practitioners are more available and more recognized now than they used to be. Magazines, periodicals, and books have increased awareness of options. Articles about the efficacy of prayer make headlines.

Much healing work is being done today through what are now called "complementary practices" or "alternative medicine." These practices treat the person through various forms of intervention including the regulation of human bioenergy fields.

That term, "bioenergy fields," probably needs some explanation – especially for those who tend towards skepticism about anything that can't be proven scientifically. (Later chapters offer some scientific evidence for these readers.)

I use "bioenergy fields" partly because I believe, from both my study and my experience, that all humans are energy fields. So far, detailed description in our language is limited. But traditional healing systems of civilizations all over the world, past and present, seem to recognize their existence in one way or another.

When I use the term "bioenergy fields," I do not necessarily subscribe to any of these other healing systems – though I certainly acknowledge the validity of some elements. Rather, this is a generic way of describing a reality; the human body is more than just a collection of organs and functions which, like a machine, can be dismantled and reassembled, or controlled by prescription medications.

Complementary practices include the following (for definitions, see Appendix A):

- Acupressure
- Acupuncture
- Applied Kinesiology
- Aromatherapy
- Bach Flower Remedies
- Craniosacral Therapy
- Healing Touch
- Homeopathy
- Light and Color Therapy
- Magnetic Field Therapy
- Massage
- Polarity Therapy
- Qi Gong
- Reflexology
- Reiki
- T'ai Chi
- Therapeutic Touch
- Yoga

Although most of these have historically taken place outside the church, in recent years the church has also recognized the validity of complementary healing, when it has sponsored courses in stress management, relaxation, and meditation. In some churches, Healing Touch, Therapeutic Touch, Reiki, and/or Reflexology are now offered by appointment.

Many in the secular scene who explore these practices for their own healing, or who are becoming equipped as practitioners, have opted out of organized religion. However, some who have been away from the church, perhaps for years, are finding their way back, having made a new and real connection with God through bioenergy work. They bring skills to enhance the church's healing ministry, and in some cases find support for these within the church. Other persons who have continued to attend church regularly are discovering healing techniques and bringing them into the pastoral care programs of the church.

And still others are exploring Native spirituality in their search for healing.

Rediscovering Native Healing Practices

For Native Americans of both North and South America, the art of healing is a way of life, inseparable from day-to-day existence, and closely connected to the earth. They understand all creation to contain a spirit, a life force; they experience Mother

Earth as a living, sensitive, breathing organism. The forces of creation are dynamically interwoven as a harmonious whole. Illness occurs when this balance is upset. Native healers believe the earth has what we might define today as an electromagnetic vibration helpful for removing imbalanced energy within a heal-ee. Therefore, whenever possible, healing work is done in a natural setting.

It is just as important to the Native healer to assist people in keeping well – by means of ceremony, dancing and singing – as it is to cure diseases. Through these rituals, a sense of harmony within the community is maintained or restored. The ceremonies unite each person individually with the deeper self, with others, and with the enfolding cosmos. Many healing ceremonies center around the drum, the sound of the heartbeat. The circle is a central symbol, for energy is believed to flow in circular movements. Therefore the forming of circles provides an effective way to generate energy and to direct prayer – a sharp contrast to the Western culture's square configurations and linear communication.

Native American healers develop their inborn gifts through living close to the earth. Their training includes meditation, power received in vision quest (opening up to the intention and enabling of the Spirit), along with apprenticeship and initiation. It is considered essential that a healer's life and healing practice be as one. Before a healing, healers will prepare themselves, the environment, and the one to be healed, with smoke from a sacred plant, usually sage, sweetgrass, or cedar. This plant, prayerfully gathered and dried, is burned and offered to the Four Directions.

Native healers learn to bring the self into harmony with a plant before uprooting it, to sit with the plants, to sense intuitively the oldest plant with the strongest energy, and to explain to the plant the need for its medicine. A prayer may request an essential exchange of energy, and further prayer be offered to the Creator so that the plant will release its energy and allow a needy one to be healed.

Ken Cohen, in an article entitled "Native American Healing Touch" in the Spring 1994 edition of *Bridges*, the Newsletter of the International Society for the Study of Subtle Energy and Energy Medicine (ISSSEEM), explains that in the process of being readied for healing, the healee may have gone through a preparation involving "sensory deprivation" (fasting and silence) and perhaps received the healing during what might be called "sensory overload" (drumming, dance, masks and costumes, sage or cedar incense).

He says further that Native healers have long understood that the forces flowing through the healer contact the life energy of the recipient, bringing that one's energy into balance. The healer takes for granted that a transfer of power from a spiritual source beyond the self is taking place. Native healers understand the necessity of not using any of their own power, which would cause a weakening and susceptibility to the illness being cured.

Cohen tells of the Seneca medicine man Moses Shongo, who would hold up one hand with fingers pointing to the sky, imagining healing power coming directly into him from the Creator's "light of Love." At the same time, the other hand did the healing, either with a gentle touch or without.

Non-contact touch is as common a means of treatment among Native healers as is direct bodily contact. In non-contact touch, the Native healer holds the hands about six inches above the body or on either side of the distressed area, focuses, and prays. Native American healers and healees pray before, during and after healing treatments. This brings about a feeling of mystical unity throughout.

Native methods of healing are influencing both the church and society in general. The wisdom of the Native circle, of respect for Mother Earth, of the use of herbs for health and healing, and the healing power of sacred communal rituals are being appreciated in a new way today. Some churches incorporate Native practices into Christian rituals: for example, the burning of sweetgrass for cleansing and blessing, and prayers to the Directions. Though such integration is still the exception in most mainline churches, the wisdom and depth in Native American spirituality and healing methods are being honored.

Native peoples have long understood and practiced a respect and appreciation for the gift of the Great Spirit in creation which non-Native society today is having to learn. Having exploited the earth, we recognize now the seriously damaging effects to the natural environment of what we have called "progress." We are having to learn to become the stewards of this earth that God always intended. The alternative is that if the planet dies, we die with it!

So today, we are called to pray for the healing of the earth as for ourselves, for we are inextricably connected with it in energy, and with one another in responsibility.

Finding Our Own Healing Practices

When many people hear of a healing ministry, they are likely to imagine what they see on television – a very evangelistic, emotionally and spiritually aggressive form of ministry. Televised healing services may seem unfamiliar, overwhelming, or even frightening for mainline churchgoers.

This media style of healing ministry does not usually fit with either the nature or theology of mainline churches. Yet in these ministries some people do get healed, and crutches do get thrown away, and the blind do see – not always, but sometimes. Is it lasting? We cannot know, but neither can we write off the ministry as totally ineffectual – or fake. And it stirs us to consider, if that mode is not what we want, then how will we exercise a healing ministry?

What is our style? It may be considerably less extroverted and overtly charismatic. We will probably conduct our healing ministry in an orderly, quiet way, whether informal or highly liturgical. Each of our denominations wants to affirm faith in the healing power of God in a language and style appropriate to that community, culturally and theologically. The challenge is to clarify what constitutes appropriate style, and to get about the healing ministry where and as we are.

Some feel called to rediscover the charismatic gifts of the Corinthian church and exercise them with boldness, power, and discernment. Others come to deeper belief in the power of healing prayer through the mind and understanding as they give attention to current healing research. Still others simply believe Jesus continues to heal today, and that settles the matter for them. They speak the word of healing, and trust God.

Whether our faith expression is conservative, liberal or in between, we are called to connect with the heart of Love in the universe, and to exercise the gifts of the Spirit in an intentional healing ministry following the command of Christ. Whether we express these gifts in silent focused thought, in words, or touch, we must do so with all the love of our hearts and the conviction of our faith.

The Vital Role of Faith

In the spring of 1997, terrible flooding caused severe damage and left many people homeless in several areas of the United States and Canada. A friend came back from North Dakota and told me of seeing this sign on a street in Grand Forks:

> *Help is everywhere.*
> *People are wonderful.*
> *Life is good in the midst of debris.*

Here was a statement of faith in the goodness of people and of life, a statement of gratitude and hope.

Faith has been described as belief without proof. We speak of having faith in the doctor, the treatment, the medicine, the counselor, the neighbor, or the government! The track record of each influences the degree of faith response. If they do fail to meet our expectations, we say we have "lost faith," lost our conviction that we can count on them.

I think of belief as belonging to the head, and faith to the heart. But our confidence in God is both belief and faith. The prayer experiments identified in later chapters give evidence that speaks to our minds, as did healing miracles to the crowds long ago. In Jesus, God showed us a love beyond our understanding. We are loved unconditionally and eternally. This speaks to our hearts.

Martin Luther said that "faith is a living, daring confidence in God's grace." To have faith in God is to trust in the nature and attributes of God. The writer to the Hebrews commended faith that was the *"assurance of things hoped for, the conviction of things not seen"* (Hebrews 11:1).

Faith as a Factor in Healing

In recording the healing miracles of Jesus, the physician Luke wrote of the faith of the centurion and the response of Jesus, the Great Physician. The centurion said,

> *"Only speak the word, and let my servant be healed..." When*
> *Jesus heard this he was amazed at him, and turning to the crowd*
> *that followed him, he said, "I tell you, not even in Israel have I*
> *found such faith." When those who had been sent returned to the*
> *house, they found the slave in good health.* (Luke 7:7b,9-10)

Similarly, Jesus spoke to the one of the ten lepers who came back and fell at Jesus' feet to give thanks:

> *Get up and go on your way; your faith has made you well.*
> **(Luke 17:19)**

And to the blind beggar sitting by the roadside, Jesus said,

> *Receive your sight; your faith has saved you.* (Luke 18:42)

Yet not all came to Jesus with such faith. Some came with doubt. Sometimes Jesus healed them to increase their faith; sometimes he healed simply out of compassion. Faith – wherever it comes from – activates the healing energy of God. Jesus knew this and he taught it.

We pray as we can, not as we cannot. We pray with the measure of faith that is ours. God increases our faith as we persist in praying, while leaving the outcome of our prayers to God.

Gifts of the Spirit

Readers of the New Testament letters to young churches have often noted the emphasis on the spiritual gift of love and its various expressions. Paul called these the "fruit" of the Spirit: love, joy, peace, patience, kindness, goodness, generosity, faithfulness, gentleness, self-control (Galatians 5:22-23). "Fruit" are companions to the "gifts." "Fruit" relate to who we are, our relationships and the spiritual quality of our lives. Spiritual "gifts" relate to what we do, our calling and our function in ministry.

In 1 Corinthians 12:8-11, Paul identifies nine "gifts" given to the church for the fulfillment of ministry: wisdom, knowledge, faith, healing, miracles, prophecy, discernment, tongues, and the interpretation of tongues. Other New Testament passages expand these gifts (for example, Romans 12:6-8, 1 Corinthians 12:28, Ephesians 4:11). This inventory of spiritual gifts is not intended to be exhaustive, for the gifting activity of the Holy Spirit is beyond what the human mind can imagine.

Gifts of the Spirit are given to every Christian. The gifts named are some of the particular gifts given for the building up of the church and the church's ministry in the world. Not everyone need operate each gift at the same time or in the same measure within the body of Christ, but none are denied to any who need. God does not play favorites!

All that we are enabled to be and do, in one way or another, is a gift of God. Therefore, all talents and natural gifts can be understood to be spiritual. As we develop these, we surrender them to God's service as we surrender ourselves. This is a gift of our gratitude to God.

All Gifts Are Equal in God's Sight

We need to be careful about thinking of some gifts as more important than others. When the Lowville United Church prayer group met on a wintry Sunday morning, the quiet might have allowed the members to become aware of the scrape of a shovel outside the window, as the custodian cleared and salted the icy steps. From the sanctuary might have come distant sounds of the organist and soloist practicing, or from the kitchen, the clatter of the coffee pot being prepared for the fellowship time.

Within the prayer group, gifts of discernment, faith, prophecy, and healing may have been exercised, or, on occasion, speaking in tongues in prayer. But equally important were the gifts evidenced by the other sounds in the church – helping, serving, and leading in music.

We need to acknowledge, accept, and welcome the range of gifts being stirred up in our lives. Sometimes we simply do not believe these gifts could be for us. In our free will, we can decline God's gifts. Doors will open, but we can ignore them or refuse to walk through.

For myself, I always wanted to be a teacher. I remember "playing school" as a child at my little desk, arranging my pencils and pads, cutting out pictures, poems and prayers from my Sunday School papers. As an adult, I enjoyed teaching school. I was effective and successful in that vocation. But I felt parts of me unfulfilled unless I became involved in working more directly in the mission of the church. So I served as Sunday School teacher, and in many other roles in the church, including the initiating of prayer groups in local churches, and participating in the healing ministry.

Eventually, God seemed to be calling me out of public education. I was drained of enthusiasm and energy. I did not know what I would do next. It was a time of life surrender.

Then doors started to open. The Spirit began stirring anew in me. I took some spiritual studies, as I waited to see what God wanted next. Lowville Prayer Centre evolved. Some of my gifts found new life and expression, and some gifts previously more latent than active came to the fore. I came to understand more fully that when God calls, God equips. My part was to be open and willing.

My ministry today still includes teaching, but in the area of prayer and healing.

In the ministry of healing, several spiritual gifts that Paul names in 1 Corinthians 12 operate in combination. Knowledge, wisdom, faith, and discernment are all important with gifts of healing. Also, we need to hear the prophetic word being spoken to the church today: through the healing work being done in the secular world, through the movement of the Spirit, through activation of healing gifts among us.

Two other workings of the Spirit may appear in the exercising of the healing ministry, and these we must consider.

Speaking in Tongues

Often a gift may quite suddenly begin to manifest in a person's life – with or without the intention of the individual. For example, a gift of speaking in tongues (glossolalia) may appear in a person's prayer or worship time – or in one's sleep! As Paul cautioned, this gift is primarily for the individual's own prayer and praise, and for the building up of the inner spirit. It is never to be a source of spiritual pride or divisiveness in the church.

In Christian ministry, the gift of speaking in tongues can also help in praying for another. The conscious mind is bypassed; the spirit of the other is addressed in language inspired by the Holy Spirit. However, speaking in tongues
is not necessary for prayer to be effective. Again, Paul reminds the Corinthians
that speaking in tongues is the least of the gifts to be sought. When we, with a
heart centered in Christ's love, pray sincerely and intently for God's highest
good for ourselves or another we have prayed well. That is all we need to do.

Wisdom and discernment are needed when speaking in tongues in prayer
for healing in a public setting. If it will frighten or create a barrier in the openness of the one receiving prayer, then it is not helpful, but a hindrance.

Altered State of Consciousness

There are other occasions when the power of the Spirit causes an altered state of
consciousness. When conscious awareness of one's self or environment is suspended,
as if one has fainted, this is described in spiritual terms by some as being "slain in the
Spirit." It may last for only a few moments or for a more prolonged length of time.

This can and does occur in one's own deep prayer or meditation when one
feels flooded and held in the light and love of God. One becomes insensible to
one's surroundings, and temporarily unable to move except with great effort.
Upon coming out from such experiences, there is a special, lingering sense of
God or Jesus' presence, a sense of peace and great love. There may also be
awareness of having been healed by the Spirit of some distress, or of having
received a special touch from God.

In a communal setting, where people are gathered in praise and prayer, open
to God and focused in faith, the presence of the Spirit can be especially strongly
felt and manifested. One person may come to a healing service, self-programmed
to be slain in the Spirit. Another may come determined not to allow such an
experience to happen. Both may be surprised!

We should not come expecting how God will move, but simply trusting in
God's love, goodness, reasons, and ways.

As with speaking in tongues, to experience an altered state of consciousness
when praying or receiving prayer does not mean that God loves that one more,
nor does it make one somehow more holy. It is simply an effect that may occur.

I have myself been "slain in the Spirit." The first time this happened, I was
in a home, praying with two friends. I had no idea what had happened. One
moment I was hearing their voices and then I suddenly crumpled to the floor,
as if in a faint. Fortunately these friends were knowledgeable enough of life in
the Spirit not to be alarmed, but just to leave me in God's hands. I believe now

that had this not been so, the experience may not have taken place as it did – God always acts with wisdom and in love.

At first I felt embarrassed upon "waking up." I certainly wondered what had happened to me. Was I sick? Had the room been too hot or stuffy?

My friends were willing to speak a little with me while I was resting, and we recognized together that God had been at work in me. There was no hurrying away for we knew I was not ready to go out to drive my car for a time!

The effect of this experience stayed with me for several days as a mild euphoric feeling, and a gentle but deep sense of God's presence, peace, and joy. I felt God's hand upon my life. It had been a holy moment – not an experience I readily wanted to talk about. It felt private, between God and me.

Getting Started in a Ministry of Healing

For any church to make a beginning, with no previous experience of healing ministry, can seem dismaying. We need to remember that we do not need to know everything about healing ministry to begin. We need only have our hearts there first – loving, caring hearts with which to respond to the call of Jesus and the need around us.

A pilgrim was making his way in the bitter cold of winter to the Himalayan mountains. An innkeeper said to him, "How will you ever get to your destination in this kind of weather?"

Replied the pilgrim cheerfully, "My heart got there first, so it's easy for the rest of me to follow."

Without doubt, this is the time for the church to move in the healing aspect of its mission. There is today an opportunity to meet people on the edges who, because of their need, are open to receiving healing through the church. This must, of course, never be a manipulation to draw people into the church, but a means to express the love of God, and the ministry of Christ in its fullness. This is the time to share the blessing of healing with one another in the church, in our families, among friends and strangers.

As with our ways of worship, our ways of healing will differ among churches and religious groups. Mainline denominations are not likely to pursue the styles seen on television or in fundamentalist crusade ministries. But in whatever form these healing ministries eventually appear, the call to minister healing is being heard.

The Spirit is stirring up the mainline church today to take up its healing mandate. And we are among those being stirred, or the three of us would not be writing this book, and you would not be reading it!

For specific examples of how some congregations have made a response to God's stirring up of the ministry of healing in their midst, see Appendix F.

Medical, Religious, and Mystical Cooperation

It's an exciting day in which we live! Theologians, mystics, scientists, doctors, and therapists are starting to talk to each other again! In past years, when intervention for healing was needed, a person's spirit, psyche, and body were treated as unrelated. The body was turned over to medical doctors, the mind and the emotions to psychiatrists and counselors, and the spirit to the clergy. We became fragmented as persons and as caring agencies.

Today, theologians are looking seriously at scientific research on the most effective ways to pray, and at recent consciousness theory. The church is being challenged to integrate into its practice a new awareness of the spiritual interconnection that exists between us, and all others, and creation. We are being called to recognize the "nonlocality" of mind (that is, that mind is not completely localized in brains, nor are bodies localized in space or present time).

This nonlocality has implications for prayer. While many doctors have no doubt always prayed for their patients, today there are doctors praying openly at bedsides as well as privately. Because of the scientific research being done around prayer, some doctors are attending more to the power of prayer as treatment.

A medical doctor, Larry Dossey, predicts in his book *Healing Words* that the "the soul-like quality of human beings" will no longer be just a declaration of religions, held by faith alone. It will be considered a "legitimate implication of rational, empirical science." He says that awareness of the "soul-like quality," the nonlocal aspect of us that does not die, will create a bridge between science and religion which will help to heal the antipathy long existing between these two.

Amazing as it may seem, science today is affirming the existence of soul or spirit, and religious communities are beginning to do energy-based healing. And nurses are working within religious communities as part of a parish's professional staff. Mystics are no longer considered to be strange people who only live on mountain tops, or in ashrams, but may be any of us journeying on the spiritual path. Encounters with the Divine (mystical experiences) are increasingly regarded as a norm of the spiritual journey. More people are meditating and are connecting with God through this means.

Whatever we, as companions on the Christian journey, can do to support and participate in this ongoing interdisciplinary dialogue will further human healing and honor the life we have together.

Science has generally been skeptical, if not downright hostile,
towards anything to do with prayer and healing.
But much of that reaction has to do with the unwillingness of
scientists to consider upsetting new concepts.
Wayne Irwin *documents the growing body of evidence about*
the efficacy of prayer and healing.

4

Pushing Back the "Boggle Threshold"

One of my hobbies is spending time with my portable short-wave radio. On one recent evening, there was much static and sputter. Then came intelligible sound – from far around the world, the unmistakable accent of a reader for the BBC World Service. "Jacques Villeneuve has just won the Hungarian Grand Prix," he announced.

But consider the chain of events leading to my hearing that announcement. In Hungary, Villeneuve had crossed the finish line. A television camera had registered the visible event. That signal had been beamed to a satellite in stationary orbit 25,000 miles above the earth, to be reflected to Great Britain. The information was carried at the speed of light by cable to a newsroom, where the story was manually keyed into a computer. A human voice read that story into a microphone in a studio. The varying frequencies and pitches of the voice were translated once more into an electronic signal superimposed on the frequencies of the 49-meter band used by the BBC that evening to broadcast its information service to North America. My portable receiver in Canada translated the signal back into audible British English. The sounds passed to a loudspeaker, into the air, into my eardrums. I recognized the language – it could, after all, have been Swahili, not English – and decoded the message, which influenced me.

If I had tried to explain to someone who did not already know about these things the incredible route that information took reaching me, that person would be totally baffled. It would boggle that person's mind. To a person living in Jesus' day, without question, it would have been termed "a miracle." Yet had the know-how and the equipment been available, the transmission would have worked in the same way it works today. Electromagnetic frequencies existed back then, even though it would be many centuries before they would be recognized.

The capability to transmit information electronically was not invented. It was discovered. But until the scientific revolution and Marconi's subsequent discovery of how to make it work, no one would believe that it was possible.

Much the same is true, I suggest, about the miracles of healing. The capacity has been there all along; but we are only now beginning to understand how it can happen.

Things We Don't Understand

Each of us has our own perception of reality. Most of the time, we hardly give a passing thought to what we know, and how we know it. When we switch on the radio, we don't care how it works. When we turn on the television, we know the persons we see are not really inside the box. We are normally only interested in the information, the music, or the feelings the program induces.

This indifference is very much like our nonchalance about ultimate reality. We rarely exercise our minds much about eternal truths and divine justice until some occurrence takes us to the edge of human experience. Then we want some answers. And the description of reality that fills our need in this new situation may bear little resemblance to the view of the nature of things that satisfied us up to that hour.

The world of science has gone through, and is going through, that kind of transformation.

Everything in the 18th and 19th centuries made sense according to the ideas and theories of 17th century Isaac Newton. Everything seemed in order. Everything seemed predictable. Science officially believed that we were close to the end of discovery, that everything that could be known was already within view.

Then, early in the 20th century, Albert Einstein posed some questions that had never before been asked. The new description of reality that these questions precipitated surpassed the "boggle threshold" of most scientists. Acceptance of the idea that the nature of the physical universe was much more mysterious than previously believed took place only slowly, with much resistance and complaining.

We Don't Expect Our Worldview to Change

Like those scientists, most of us expect to live out our lives within a stable conceptual framework. We presume our understanding of reality will remain relatively constant, as it did for our parents and their parents and their grand-parents long before. It gives us a familiar lens through which we view and interpret whatever happens.

This accepted view of reality allows us to live without having to re-examine our basic assumptions anew each day. We live within a particular culture, in a certain family; we are raised within a specific religion, are all taught the same basic rules, and introduced to the same fundamental norms of understanding, so that each invisible component of our societal structure can function in an efficient equilibrium. This worldview, or "paradigm" as it is called, becomes a filter through which each experience is automatically sifted to determine whether it fits our framework of life.

If an experience cannot pass through that filter, it is usually discarded, discounted, and considered nonfactual, not real.

The Worldview of the Local Church
Affects its Healing Ministry

These worldviews greatly affect the possibility of a healing ministry within a congregation. And that congregation's view of reality is influenced severely by the local culture. People's minds and expectations place limits upon what can be expected, and interfere with outcomes that would otherwise be possible.

Much of the present worldview of the church is based, not on concepts taught by Jesus and the early church, but on philosophies and theologies that have gained sway since. We declare ourselves to be Presbyterians or Lutherans, Calvinists or Barthians, proponents of feminist or evangelical theology. And sometimes we lose touch with our primary allegiance.

Much of our prevailing theology, for example, comes not from the Bible but from St. Augustine. His roots were in the dualistic theology of Manichaeism and the philosophy of Neoplatonism. He found the Bible "unintelligible and full of crudities," although he found some "reasonableness" in the writings of St. Paul. Most of Augustine's teaching had little reference to Jesus at all. And yet, because of the politics of the Empire at the time, his thought became the official theology of Rome. Heresy became a crime, punishable by death. He formulated the first Christian theory of the "just war."

And he taught that God created the world *ex nihilo* – from nothing – and that God then stepped back, choosing to remain aloof, to avoid enmeshing the Sacred Nature in the profanity of the created order. This was not biblical; but, until recently, the Western church accepted Augustine's view uncritically.

So the church has tended to imply in its teaching that we are here on earth, and that God is somewhere else – presumably in heaven – ignoring the biblical affirmation that even heaven is part of the created order. Liturgies used in worship often use the words: "May God be with you." For the untrained hearer, the words convey an implication that God is sometimes not. One man, in a workshop that Flora and I conducted, stated plainly that he did his talking with God in the morning and the evening, but that during his working day he figured he was "on his own."

I don't claim this is a universal attitude. I merely point out that if a church believes that God is not already present, but must be invoked – called in – it will have a different task of education to perform in preparing for a healing ministry than a church that believes that God is always near.

Many Hold the Traditional Scientific Worldview

The traditional scientific worldview which permeates our Western culture, if it allows for the concept of God at all, puts forward this same philosophy. If God exists, it is only as the Prime Mover, the First Cause. There is no involvement anymore. Once the clockwork was wound up, God withdrew.

This is not, we should notice, the view that was taught by Jesus and by the writers of the biblical record. Jesus stressed the unity of God with present experience. In John 10:30, Jesus says to the Jews gathered in the temple,

The Father and I are one.

In John 14:20, he says to his disciples,

I am in my Father, and you in me, and I in you.

In Matthew 28:20, he says,

Remember, I am with you always.

This understanding of God being with us, being always accessible to us, never far from us, is the biblical view. Some favorite words from the Psalms affirm it:

> *Where can I go from your spirit?*
> *Or where can I flee from your presence?*
> *If I ascend to heaven, you are there;*
> *if I make my bed in Sheol, you are there.*
> *If I take the wings of the morning*
> *and settle at the farthest limits of the sea,*
> *even there your hand shall lead me,*
> *and your right hand shall hold me fast.* (Psalm 139:7ff)

The apostle Paul refers to it in his speech in Athens to the assembled politicians at Mars Hill:

> *God is not far from each one of us.* (Acts 17:27)

The Dominant Western Worldview

Like all societies, our modern Western world is organized around a dominant central understanding of reality. It goes something like this:

> *Long ago, everything in the universe was contained in one*
> *compact very hot ball – a cosmic egg – so small*
> *that it was only a point. Nothing else existed.*
> *And somehow, this egg exploded, and this "big bang" was such*
> *that matter and space began expanding in every direction.*
> *After something like 15 billion years of evolution*
> *of star galaxies and solar systems,*
> *there came together on the planet Earth*
> *certain chemicals that resulted in life.*
> *Then came further development of ever-more complex life forms,*
> *following certain "laws of natural selection."*
> *Increasingly intricate formations of neural networking culminated*
> *in the formation of the human brain with its astonishing capabili-*
> *ties. The essential characteristics of human nature were the*
> *consequence of a succession of random events – accidental,*
> *without purpose or meaning. The essence of our personal identity*

*is found in the DNA which informs our development. Our basic
drives are survival, pleasure, and procreation.*

*The primary guide to our decision making is economic logic and
values. The Earth and our fellow inhabitants are "resources" to be
used in the service of the economy. Our crowning achievement is
our ability to control nature by means of technology.*

Nothing exists beyond the visible physical world.

And death is the end.

We Are Not the Only Conscious Life Forms

Recently, some discoveries have been made that shake that worldview as much
as Albert Einstein's Theory of Relativity shook the Newtonian worldview of the
18th and 19th centuries.

In 1966, Cleve Backster was working in the office of his lie detector school
in New York City. On an impulse, he attached the electrodes of one of his lie
detectors to a large tropical plant in the room. He wondered if the leaves
would indicate any measurable response when the plant had water poured
on its roots. Indeed, there was a reaction, similar to an emotional response in
a human being.

Backster was intrigued. Knowing that the most effective way to make the
reading jump with a human subject was to threaten the person's well-being, he
decided to irritate the plant. He dunked one of its leaves in his hot coffee. No
reaction. He waited a moment, deciding next to light a match and burn the leaf
to which his electrodes were attached. Even before he could reach for a match,
the machine indicated a reaction. Backster had made no move yet. But it seemed
that the plant had sensed his plan.

Further testing indicated that the plant was able to distinguish between genuine intention and "just pretend."

As Backster continued his whimsical pursuit, he found that plants with which
he had some sort of personal connection would react even when he was 15
miles away. Any plant that he selected in his mind to be destroyed would respond by entering what he described as an "altered state of consciousness."
They would "pass out" – wilt.

He later demonstrated to a group of scientists at Yale that even the movements of a spider in the same room would cause a reaction in the leaf. Again,
the response occurred just before the spider moved, as if the plant could sense
spider intentions.

Five years later, Marcel Vogel, a research chemist with IBM, began experiments based on this so-called "Backster Effect." He examined the affinity between plants and humans, and between plants and other plants. He learned that if he attached two plants to the same galvanometer, when a leaf was snipped from one, the other would respond to the hurt. But the second plant only seemed to do so when he was paying attention to it. Vogel described this phenomenon by an analogy of two lovers. He said it seemed as though he and the second plant were connected emotionally at the heart, until one of them (himself) became distracted. Then the flow of information was blocked.

He wondered whether the second plant was actually reacting to the pain of the first, or whether it was reading him.

We Discount Unexpected Occurrences as "Anomalies"

Others attempted to replicate Vogel's work, conscientiously striving to eliminate any possibility of a heart connection. They observed no response – perhaps because that was the result they wanted.

Many biologists subsequently breathed a sigh of relief, dismissing it all as unworthy of consideration. There are many, in every field, who shy away from anomalies – happenings that do not fit their theories. Persons who have invested their life in a certain understanding of reality have no interest in rearranging their mental furniture. Even theologians have a vested interest in their fundamental worldview not being changed.

Any of us, if something seems to challenge our understanding of reality, have a tendency to reject the new information. We discount the experience, interpret it all as a mistaken observation, or treat it as a mystery that simply has an unknown but still conventional explanation. We are extremely resistant to any threat to our worldview. And so we should be; for it is foundational to our handling of life.

Nevertheless, we know that we must countenance change, from time to time, because change itself is a part of how we have come to where we are. Basic change, however, is never initiated by orthodoxy. And it proceeds only when there is a universal shift in the basic assumptions undergirding life.

Such a universal shift is taking place today.

Plants Can Apparently Talk to Each Other

For thousands of years, we have treated plants as the lowest form of life. They were alive, yes, but they could not move. We assumed, therefore, that they could not think, or communicate, or feel pain or joy.

Today, it is clear that plant life also has a consciousness, and that one tree can actually communicate to another.

In the northwestern Transvaal, in Africa, large numbers of kudu – a spiral-horned antelope – were apparently starving. But there were plenty of leaves at hand. Wouter van Hoven, a physiologist from the University of Pretoria, came to investigate. He noted that the leaves the kudu were eating contained enough protein for the animals' well-being, but the animal droppings retained far more protein than they should. The food was not being properly digested.

Upon further analysis, the reason for the kudu demise became evident. The van Hoven team found that the leaves contained chemical compounds known as "tannins" – insoluble compounds used, for example, in tanning leather to protect it against micro-organisms. The tannins from the leaves, in the kudu stomachs, similarly prevented digestive microbes from doing their job.

Biologist Lyall Watson, in *The Nature of Things*, explains that as animals have found plants to eat, plants invented defenses. Heavy bark and thorns are obvious physical deterrents. There are also chemical deterrents. Some make the plants taste bitter, others make them poisonous.

In this case, the thornbush deterred browsing by producing tannins in their leaves that made the taste change rapidly. As a result, the kudu would normally browse briefly at one tree, and then move on. But because new fences in the area restricted the animals from wandering as far as normal, the kudu were being forced to feed more often than usual from the same trees.

Van Hoven's researchers found that the trees produced the extra chemical within minutes. After only 15 minutes, the concentration of tannin would rise in some trees by 44 percent, in others by as much as 94 percent. After an hour, the level would be up over 250 percent. And it would take a full day, and in some cases more than three days, for the plants to return to their relaxed and normal state.

The team also observed that nearby trees from which no leaves had yet been eaten also showed a measurable increase in tannins. These other trees were not simply responding to an attack on themselves – here was clear evidence of actual communication of danger between plants, not in a laboratory but in the wilds.

Our Basic Assumptions about Life Are Being Stretched

Most people resist such ideas because they begin to stretch our basic assumptions about life. They challenge us with the possibility that the central myth that has served Western society for so many generations is inadequate.

We in the church, as declared followers of Jesus, desiring to reclaim and redevelop his healing ministry, need to resist being followers of the world. Rather than clinging to this outdated understanding, we need to turn intentionally to the reported words of Jesus to get in touch with the understanding of reality that we need.

Jesus' view of reality was a basic philosophy of "connectedness." We find it constantly in his familiar words:

> *Just as you did it to one of the least of these who are*
> *members of my family, you did it to me.*
> (Matthew 25:40).
> *You have heard that it was said, "You shall love your neighbor*
> *and hate your enemy." But I say to you, Love your enemies*
> *and pray for those who persecute you,*
> *so that you may be children of your Father in heaven.*
> (Matthew 5:43-45a)
> *I am the vine, you are the branches.*
> *Those who abide in me and I in them bear much fruit,*
> *because apart from me you can do nothing.*
> (John 15:5)

North America Learns from Other Cultures

When James Reston of *The New York Times* needed surgery during a trip to Beijing in 1971, the Chinese used Western-style surgery. But they also inserted three slender acupuncture needles into his knees and right elbow to relieve his postoperative pain.

The Chinese have lived for millennia with an understanding of reality in which acupuncture is known and accepted. But until Reston reported it, it was little known in our culture. Although it has since become commonplace here too, the first use of acupuncture for anesthesia took place in 1972 in the United States. Anesthesiologist John W. C. Fox, of Brooklyn, used four fine-gauge needles on a medical student undergoing surgery for the removal of a growth on his tonsils. The needles were inserted in the webbing between the thumb and forefinger of each hand, and in the skin between the second and third toes of each foot.

Since then, acupuncture has become well established within Western practice. It is also being used successfully today, for example, for persons recovering from heroin addiction. Our editor has a young friend who tried for years, unsuccessfully, to quit smoking. Acupuncture enabled him to succeed.

The Search for a Conventional Explanation

Originally, Western culture scoffed at acupuncture's principle of "meridians" running through the body. But in the 1960s, Korean medical researchers used microdissection methods to seek a conventional explanation for acupuncture. They found evidence of an independent series of ducts, unrelated to the vascular and lymphatic systems known to the West. They observed that fluids did flow within these tubes. And in a study published in 1985, French researcher Pierre de Vernejoul, having injected radioactive isotopes and tracked their movement, verified the existence of the "meridian system." Numerous tests to measure the galvanic skin response of acupuncture points found that they had higher electrical conductance than surrounding skin. Under a grant from the American National Institutes of Health, researcher Robert Becker showed that electrical currents flowed along these channels. He and his colleagues reasoned that the points acted like repeater stations to boost the signals as they traveled along the meridians, and that the insertion and spinning of a needle would interfere with that flow.

In Japan, researcher Hiroshi Motoyama developed a computerized device for measuring the functions of the meridians and diagnosing physiological imbalances. Its technology is now being used by some medical practitioners in the West, particularly for research into Parkinson's Disease. This diagnostic tool clearly correlates the status of deep internal organs with the ancient Chinese theory associating particular meridians with specific organ systems.

Acupuncture, in other words, long derided by Western medicine as fakery or as autosuggestion, has now been shown by Western scientific experimental methods to have its own validity. It raises the possibility – even the likelihood – that other non-Western insights may also have a scientific basis.

The Chinese Understanding of "Life Energy"

The Eastern understanding of connectedness is central to the theories of *Qi Gong*.

Traditional Chinese medicine holds that a person is a unity within which illness results from an imbalance between the flow of "life energy" and the fluids of the body. The Chinese call the energy *Qi* or *chi* – pronounced "chee." (You may have heard the word in "T'ai Chi" exercise programs.) They express this imbalance in terms of a negative energy (yin) and a positive energy (yang).

Qi Gong combines meditation, body movement, and breath regulation to influence the flow of this life energy. Practicing it has been shown to lower blood pressure, metabolic rate, and level of dopamine – the enzyme that controls activ-

ity of the brain. Developed over thousands of years, the practice of Qi Gong includes sensitivity to the time of day and the time of year when certain exercises
are most beneficial. It is tied to the natural rhythms of the planet. Practices have
been passed down through individual families, resulting in thousands of variations. It is also known to be extremely effective in prevention of problems. It has
even been a means for individuals essentially to heal themselves of serious illness.

The Toxins that Afflict Us

Western medicine has made vast strides since the days when doctors kept boxes
of leeches in their offices, to bleed away a person's "bad blood." But despite this
progress, the conventional understanding of disease is actually a theory. An im-
mense industry of medicine and pharmacy has been assembled upon that theory.
There are powerful economic reasons as to why that view will only slowly yield.

And yet the conventional view is not the only theory. One of the great clas-
sics of health literature, which orthodoxy has largely ignored, is John H. Tilden's
Toxemia Explained.

Tilden was a 19th century American physician who began to question the
use of medication as a universal remedy for illness. His extensive study led him
to conclude that there should be some way to live so as not to build disease.
During this period, he began to formulate a theory about toxemia. From the
beginning of his Denver practice, he used no medicines. Instead, he worked to
cleanse the body of its toxins, followed by lifestyle changes to allow the body to
be restored to health. He had marvelous results.

Tilden viewed every disease as a crisis of toxemia – self-poisoning – manifested in various ways. The toxin accumulates in the blood above a toleration
point, precipitating the crisis. It may appear as headache or cold, as flu or fever.
Each of these is actually the body's attempt to cure itself by eliminating the overload of toxins that the body has been unable to handle normally. Any treatment,
such as medicines, may obstruct this cleansing effort and complicate the problem. Cancer, in Tilden's view, is the culmination of years of toxemia from im-
proper nutrition and faulty elimination, caused not so much by an individual's
choices as by society's habits.

The source of every disease, Tilden suggested, is "enervation." The proper
general treatment is fasting and quiet rest. Given the chance, he claimed, the
body knows what to do to restore health. As for germs, Tilden viewed them
more as symptom than cause. Even germs, he argued, are necessary to health.

Clearly Tilden's view differs from conventional belief.

An Ancient Theory of "Vitalism" Returns

Centuries ago, it was postulated that the power which governed both health and disease was something termed "vitalism." It was thought to be an animating force which entered the organism at the time of conception, directed all the functions of life, and departed at the time of death. Paracelsus, the Renaissance alchemist and physician reported that it radiated from one person to another. The 17th century Flemish chemist and physician, van Helmont, declared that this vital force enabled one person to affect another at a distance. And the German chemist, Baron von Reichenbach, asserted that the energy could be stored, and that substances could contain it. Those who affirmed its existence believed that it was the connecting link between the individual and the universe.

Harold Saxton Burr, in *Fields of Life*, published in 1972, reported on his systematic research into bioelectric fields. Over a period of 30 years, he studied organisms, from single cells to human beings, showing that every living system possesses "an electrical field of great complexity, which can be shown to have correlations with growth and development, degeneration and regeneration, and the orientation of component parts in the whole system."

While Burr was doing his investigations, Semyon and Valentina Kirlian, in Russia, were using "Kirlian photography" (high-voltage photography) to capture the electrodynamic field permeating and surrounding the object. Their dramatic pictures excited researchers everywhere. Subsequently, countless such photographs have been published in books and magazines, showing visually that the identity of an object is not bounded by its skin.

Kirlian photography forces us to consider the question: "If who I am is not limited by my physical perimeter, then where do 'I' stop and 'you' begin?"

Romanian physician Ion Dumitrescu has gone even further. He developed a technique called "electrographic imaging" which visually represents electrical resistance just above the surface of the skin. Some call the phenomenon "electroluminescence." Bright or dark areas around acupuncture points clearly identify specific needs within the body for healing work.

Harry Oldfield and Roger Coghill in England are currently pursuing experiments based on these bioelectrical perceptions. They have already found that one of the strands of the DNA helix acts as a transmitter, the other as a receiver, and that disease is a sort of electronic warfare in which these "radios" have become "tuned out" and are no longer receiving their proper instructions from the brain. Ultraviolet radiation is sometimes known to cause this kind of interference at such a basic physical level. They postulate that remission in cancer may be the result of these "radios" becoming "tuned in" again.

Gandhi Understood Jesus' Worldview

Gandhi – called "Mahatma," meaning "Great Soul" – was a follower of the philosophy of Hinduism. But Gandhi nevertheless acknowledged the great value of Jesus' teachings, meditating each day on a portion of the Sermon on the Mount.

One day, Gandhi was rushing to catch a train. Since it was already moving, he was pushed forward by those who had brought him to the station, and pulled onto a car by those already on board. In the scramble, he lost a sandal. Once on board, he reached down, removed his other sandal, and threw it out the door.

His retinue, baffled, asked, "Gandhi, why did you do that?"

His reply testified to his understanding of connectedness. "You see," he said, "in a little while a poor man will come walking along the tracks. He will see a sandal that is of no use to him. Now, a little further along, he will find another one, and go back for the first. If I had not done what I did, I would possess one useless sandal, and so would he."

We are all connected, even across traditional lines of religious philosophy.

How the Body Processes Information

It is important for us not to be afraid of ideas simply because they come from other cultures or religions. In fact, it benefits those of us involved in healing ministry within the Christian church to have some familiarity with certain understandings from Gandhi's philosophical heritage, from Indian yogic theory. People ask about these things.

In contemporary society in the West, there has been much recent reference to the *chakras* of the body (Sanskrit for "wheels"), and to the principles of Ayurvedic medicine. The writings of medical doctor Deepak Chopra, trained in both traditions, have popularized these terms. According to Indian science, chakras are the way the body transmits and receives "subtle information." They act like transformers, stepping down the frequencies of the subtle information coming in, and stepping up the subtle information going out. There seem to be more than 360 chakras, corresponding with various locations in the body where acupuncture's meridians cross. Here, Chinese and Indian understandings coincide.

Each major chakra is associated with a major nerve plexus and a major endocrine gland. Each is also connected with a specific type of extrasensory sensing (that is, sensing by means beyond the five traditional senses: hearing, seeing, smelling, tasting, and touching). For example, the brow chakra, associated with the forehead, is often called "the third eye." It relates to the pituitary gland, the master gland of the endocrine system.

Indian philosophy identifies seven major chakras. They form a vertical line, ascending in complexity from the base of the spine to the top of the head. According to the Indian understanding, they connect to each other by fine threads of energetic matter known as *nadis* – channels of life energy – different from the meridians of the Chinese system. Tradition describes up to 72,000 nadis in the subtle anatomy of the human being. Because of their interconnection with the nervous system, any chakra dysfunction will have a detrimental effect upon the functioning of the body.

The ancient tantric yoga literature metaphorically represents these whirlpool-like flows of energy as flowers, with each petal of the chakra (actually each "wheel within a wheel") identified with a specific human emotion. For example, the "fear" petal is in the pit of the stomach. Furthermore, each of these petals responds to a pitch and frequency for intoning one of the letters of the Sanskrit language. Each letter corresponds to one petal. This tradition independently corroborates the experiments of Western biomusicologists, who have developed therapies based on glandular secretions in response to certain sounds.

Eastern and Western Research

Research in Japan, again by Motoyama, has tended to confirm this chakra system. And Valerie Hunt, of the University of California at Los Angeles (UCLA), has measured bioelectrical energy variations on the skin surface in the location of these chakras. She has found high-frequency oscillations never before reported in scientific literature. Normal brain waves can range as high as 100 cycles per second, although the average is under 30. Muscle frequency rises to about 225, with the heart muscle managing up to 250. She found readings in the vicinity of the chakras ranging up to 1,600 cycles per second, far above what was traditionally expected. And other tests suggested these were only lower harmonics of even higher frequencies of subtle energy moving through the chakras.

Since each chakra is understood to be tuned to a different frequency, each is presumably able to access the specific appropriate information available from the surrounding "universal energy field." This information is received, it is believed, by means of what some call "the ray," which enters through the top of the head, and is "broadcast" through the body – each area, each cell, tuning in to the specific guidance that it needs.

Connectedness Not Restricted to Human Life

This concept may well test your "boggle threshold." Given our traditional views of medicine, of science, and of how the world works, it may be hard for many of us to credit.

But there is indeed widespread evidence that even the most primitive of organisms can tune in to some kind of guidance. Harvard researcher Herbert Benson described an experiment on the ability of marine sponges to assemble and reassemble themselves. Marine sponges consist of several different types of cells, gathered around supporting skeletons. These cells work together so closely, and in such consistent form, that these cellular aggregations are classified as distinct individuals and given recognized scientific classifications. Any such group can be taken from the ocean floor, cut up, and squeezed through silk cloth so fine that it separates every cell from its neighbor. And yet, Benson found, if this formless porridge is allowed to stand quietly for a while, it soon reorganizes itself into the complete sponge again – impossible to distinguish from the original.

In one such experiment, a red sponge classified as *microciona prolifera* and a yellow *cliona celata* sponge were sieved together and their cells thoroughly mixed. But after just 24 hours, the red and the yellow cells had successfully separated themselves, reorganized, and reassembled themselves, getting back together as a red sponge and a yellow sponge.

The experiment raises awesome questions about identity. If two distinct living organisms existed at the beginning, then who was who, and who was alive and who was dead, in the blended soup? The individual cells were clearly living, but was the organism, the sponge? And if the sponge was dead, how did the cells know to reassemble themselves?

Sheldrake's New Understanding of Biology

In 1981, biologist Rupert Sheldrake staggered the scientific establishment. His book, *A New Science of Life,* was a body blow to the ensconced worldview. One of Great Britain's leading scientific magazines, *Nature,* in an anonymous editorial, vilified it as "the best candidate for burning there has been for many years." This emotional response was clear evidence of a conceptual shift in what constitutes a threat to the well-being of society.

In the book, Sheldrake attempted to address two unsolved questions:
- What is the nature of life itself?
- How are the instructions concerning the form of an organism imparted?

His answer was a revolutionary hypothesis. Sheldrake postulated that all organisms, including human beings, are formed and shaped by the energy fields surrounding and interpenetrating them.

There are two parts to the theory, Sheldrake said.

First, there is the concept of the field itself. Each organism has within it and around it a field, in the same way that a magnet has a field. But rather than being radiated by the organism, this "morphogenetic field" is an organizing field.

Second, the concept of "morphic resonance" determines how organisms relate to one another. Sheldrake noted that nature has several different kinds of fields: gravitational, electromagnetic, the strong and the weak fields of quantum physics, as well as quantum matter fields, and electron fields. None of these are reducible into each other; they are distinct. In his view, his morphic fields are as fundamental to life as any of the others. He described a morphic field as a way of conceptualizing how a particular crystal, animal, or plant would tune in to all the previous beings of its kind, across time and space.

By implication, then, a morphic field is not limited to the immediate time frame.

In 1990, researchers at Nottingham University in Great Britain began an experiment to test Sheldrake's hypothesis, using crossword puzzles. They reasoned that if morphic resonance was genuine, then it would be easier to solve today's *London Evening Standard* crossword puzzle tomorrow because other people had already solved it today. They were able to clearly show that people did indeed find the puzzle easier to solve the day after. Somehow the persons working on the puzzle tuned in to those who had worked on it the day before.

Other tests were also run with similar results, stimulated by a competition organized by the Institute of Noetic Sciences in Sausalito, California.

Since then, Sheldrake has continued to develop his theory. One model suggests that the whole of the past is in some sense present everywhere, and that organisms can tune in to everything in it. Another involves the idea of a resonant transmission taking place through other dimensions or through other realms of being. A third picks up on physicist David Bohm's controversial theories, suggesting that this morphic resonance depends on connections beyond time and space altogether. A fourth model proposes that morphic resonance has a lot in common with "quantum nonlocality," a theory now generally accepted by quantum physicists, which describes a mysterious connection that remains between subatomic particles that have separated from each other.

The "Web of Life"

All of this research – whether or not one grants it credibility – implies a vast and interconnected "web of life."

The idea of this web is not new. It has been spoken of through the ages as the interdependence of all things. When Suquamish Chief Seattle was required to transfer his tribal lands to the arriving people of the United States, he spoke of this connectedness:

> *The earth does not belong to man, man belongs to the earth.*
> *All things are connected like the blood which unites us all.*
> *Man did not weave the web of life, he is merely a strand in it.*
> *Whatever he does to the web, he does to himself.*

The "Organizing Fields" of the Body

And this brings us back to the Indian chakras.

Jack Schwarz, an American pioneer in psycho-physiological research, makes a careful distinction in his book *Human Energy Systems* between incoming and outgoing information. If we think of the ray as the input, as the incoming current, then, says Schwartz, we can think of the human aura as primarily the output, or the emanation.

Though not all of us have seen an "aura," we have all experienced the sensation of having our "privacy zone" invaded by someone unwelcome moving in too close.

Barbara Ann Brennan, a former research scientist for NASA, and founder of the Barbara Brennan School of Healing, describes the human aura in *Hands of Light.* The interwoven energies of the aura are detectable by sight or touch, with some perceptible only in an altered state of consciousness. She speaks of these fields as expanding beyond the physical body, like the auras made visible in Kirlian photography. Each of the major chakras has its own particular band of frequencies.

The ray, Schwartz says, contains all our potentials; the aura mainly reveals what we are experiencing or have experienced. Flora told me of a conversation she had with a healer who reportedly could easily see the colors of another's aura. As they talked, the healer unexpectedly interrupted Flora: "Did what I just said make you angry?"

Flora admitted, "Yes, it did."

The healer explained, "I saw a flash of red streak through your aura."

Research Continues to Offer Support

William Tiller of Stanford University has been working to apply scientific models to explain these mind-boggling concepts. He observes that most systems in the universe display entropy – the tendency to decay, disintegrate, and become less organized. Living systems, on the other hand, display the opposite. They tend to come into greater order, greater complexity.

Tiller hypothesizes that the formerly imaginary concept of "negative space/time" may well apply to life itself. In negative space/time, information moves faster than the speed of light, and thought forms charged with emotional intensity can actually linger. He believes that astral energies may operate at speeds as high as 10^{20} (1 followed by 20 zeros) times the speed of light.

Daniel Benor, American psychologist, speaking at the 2nd Conference of ISSSEEM (the International Society for the Study of Subtle Energy and Energy Medicine), thinks that the brain is a transducer for the soul. Our personal distinctiveness, he suggested, is affected by the circuitry of the brain. But it does not originate in the brain.

The more one is involved in healing, Benor says, the more it appears that consciousness shapes reality. There may well be levels of reality or distinct dimensions where particular natural laws apply, but we cannot be sure whether this is an objective reality or a creation of our minds.

Once we accept that we are not limited by our physical existence, he concluded, it is difficult to define where our boundaries might begin or end.

> Healers tell us that this awareness may be a gateway to the most
> important aspect of what healing offers, a sense of spirituality,
> which our natural culture has discouraged us from believing in or
> engaging in.

A New Worldview Is Emerging

These ways of thinking about connectedness, about organizing fields and patterns, about information, about process and change, are becoming incorporated into a new worldview that is already beginning to supplant the existing one as surely as the ideas of Déscartes and Newton deposed older views.

But many of us are afraid of such significant change, because we fear the unknown. 'Twas ever thus, it seems. In Jesus' time, the status quo felt safe, familiar. The scribes and Pharisees were not prepared to let the new ideas of this Jesus succeed. Even the people in his own home town were closed to him:

"Where did this man get this wisdom, and these deeds of power?"
they asked. "Is not this the carpenter's son?"
(Matthew 13:54b-55a)

So it is in our own day. To change the basic paradigm is to unsettle everything, to move things from the assumed state of equilibrium. The fear that arises expresses the apprehension, the concern, that the new state may not be better than the old, and may not be reversible. It is a primal fear. Without trust in the reality of the resurrection power of the Divine, it is an aspect of the universal fear of death.

The bottom line of the dominant Western world view is that "Death is the end." As theologian William Stringfellow, in *Instead of Death*, eloquently defined it:

> *Death is the power that abrasively addresses us with the word that*
> *we are not only eventually and finally estranged, separated,*
> *alienated, lost in relationships with everybody and*
> *everything else at once, but even now and already.*

In the dominant worldview of Western society, Stringfellow says, death means total loss of identity. Such is certainly the view of all entangled in the traditional scientific understanding of reality. Sadly, many within the church hold this view.

But the Christian faith affirms that death is *not* the end! The end, revealed in the resurrection of Jesus, is *life* – a new consciousness and identity at home in the heart of God. None other than Einstein said,

> *We, as human beings, are part of the whole*
> *that we call the universe, a part limited in time and space.*
> *We experience ourselves, our thoughts and feelings,*
> *as something separated from the rest – a kind of optical illusion*
> *from our consciousness. This illusion is a prison for us,*
> *restricting us to our personal desires*
> *and to affection for only the few people nearest us.*
> *Our task must be to free ourselves from this prison by*
> *widening our circle of compassion*
> *to embrace all living beings and all of nature.*

Those who are involved in healing ministry within the church are, of course, a part of that wider universe. Our motivation is not fear, but freedom. For we have confidence that new concepts, new understandings, will confirm an interconnected universe that has already been promised to us. That confidence can scarcely be expressed in more profound terms than in the classic phrases of the prologue to John's Gospel:

> *The divine word and wisdom was there with God,*
> *and it was what God was.*
> *It was there with God from the beginning.*
> *everything came to be by means of it;*
> *nothing that exists came to be without its agency.*
> *In it was life,*
> *and this life was the light of humanity.*
> *Light was shining in the darkness,*
> *and darkness did not master it.*
> (John 1:1-5, Scholars Version)

*In the almost mystical connection that each of us has with other living beings – and indeed with the whole cosmos – we are most closely connected to our own bodies. As **Rochelle Graham** explains, each part of the body can inform us about our total well-being.*

5

The Wisdom of the Body

The physical body contains the wisdom of God; it has been created this way.

This starts with an inherent belief: we are not separate from God. In restoring wholeness, balance and harmony within ourselves and in relationship to God, our bodies will communicate to us the imbalance, the disharmony and the brokenness with which we live. Both as healers and as those seeking healing, our task is to listen deeply to the wisdom within each of us, trusting that each part of the body longs to be restored to the whole and will guide us in the restoration. We simply need to learn to translate the body's symbolic language.

This chapter introduces one model for listening to the wisdom of the body. Keep in mind that these concepts are only possibilities; the cues for each person may have a different meaning. When we listen deeply, the soul within the body will tell the story.

Our Bodies as Teacher

Our body speaks to us and teaches us through symptoms or sensations. These may be pleasurable, neutral, noxious or painful. Thomas Moore in his book *Care of the Soul* calls these symptoms the "voice of the soul." When we don't listen and respond, the feedback usually gets stronger, in several ways.

Our spoken words reveal the body's wisdom, often in symbols and figures of speech. When we again listen deeply, the clues are revealed. I recall a client coming to see me because of pain in her right leg. As we talked, the client described how she felt; she "didn't have a leg to stand on." The death of her father had left her feeling emotionally, mentally and spiritually unsupported. Her physical body mirrored this feeling and called out for attention.

Emotions and thought patterns and our soul also speak through our bodies. When we feel fear or anger, our bodies will tense. Our physiology responds in a protective manner, even if it is to a memory. Whenever we allow our thoughts to become stuck in a negative pattern, such as worrying over a possible future event, our body physiology will again respond to prepare us physiologically.

Take, for example, driving in rush hour traffic. Someone cuts in front of you; you slam on the brakes and your body responds with anger and fear. These emotions trigger an SOS signal which puts your autonomic nervous system on full alert. The brain only hears " danger, danger, danger." Your heartbeat increases and your adrenal glands flood your bloodstream with adrenalin and cortisol, the flight or fight hormones. This shuts off everything not required for the emergency; at such a time rational, reflective thought is not even possible!

Recalling such an event – or simply imagining it – can elicit a similar response.

Our spiritual self also communicates through the body. If we experience the peace and calm of spiritual well-being, our bodies respond. In a reversal of the emergency reaction, the heartbeat slows down, the autonomic nervous system moves towards relaxation. The Institute of HeartMath teaches people how to change their perception of stress and monitor their hearts to check their perception. When 28 test subjects used this technique for one month, HeartMath researchers say they achieved a 100 percent increase in DHEA, said to be an anti-aging hormone.

By understanding the function of each part of the whole body, we can begin to understand symbolically what that might mean on a physical, emotional, mental and spiritual level. The function of an organ on a physical and physiological level can help us understand how it connects on a symbolic level.

Created both Male and Female

So God created humankind in his image, in the image of God
he created them; male and female he created them. (Genesis 1: 27)

This biblical insight confirms the conclusions of psychology and of other traditions: we have both masculine and feminine qualities within us. In Jungian terms this would be described as the archetypal *animus* and *anima,* or in Chinese terms, the *yang* and the *yin.*

The right side of the body – and this applies to both sexes – is said to represent the masculine side. Any symptoms on this side of the body, then, may have to do with those aspects of our being that we think of as masculine – our aggressive, assertive, logical, and rational sides.

The right side of the body may also reflect our relationship with our inner male. For example, if a woman feels a lot of external anger at men, her right side, the masculine side of her body, may cry out with symptoms. In men, symptoms on the right side may "speak" about their own masculine side, or may symbolize their relationships with other men such as their father and grandfathers.

The left side of the body, similarly, represents the feminine energy – our creative, receptive, and intuitive side. Our bodies, whether male or female, will show symptoms if we have our emotions "packed away" or if we resist receiving. An example is a woman who came to me with lots of aches and pains, mainly on her left side. She described herself as "battered and bruised by the men in her life." She had not received any physical beating, but she felt emotionally battered. In the same way, a man who feels uncomfortable expressing the qualities that would be called feminine may find his left side crying out for expression.

When listening to the body, it is helpful to observe which side of the body displays the symptom.

The Wisdom of the Lungs and Heart

The spiritual center of our bodies is the chest. The heart, as I mentioned in chapter 1, is our point of contact with God, the unifying model for life. When God breathed the breath of life into the nostrils of the first creatures in Genesis, their lungs in their chests filled with God's spirit. This is the place where God's spirit connects with the dust of earth, our physical bodies.

Our lungs are also the place where we let go of what no longer serves us. Our lungs teach us that, minute to minute, breath to breath, our spirits need to receive and let go just as our lungs receive oxygen and let go of carbon dioxide.

Dissected, the lungs resemble a tree with all its branches. We can read Revelation 22:1-2 as an analogy of the body:

> And the angel showed me the river of the water of life,
> bright as crystal, flowing from the throne of God and
> of the Lamb through the middle of the street of the city.
> On either side of the river is the tree of life...and the leaves
> of the tree are for the healing of the nations.

The throne of God and Christ within in us is the spiritual heart center; the lungs are the tree of life.

The lungs are essential for maintaining balance in the body. Each minute, to be fully alive, we breathe deeply. When unconsciously we choose not to feel, or not to be aware of what we are feeling, we will often breathe shallowly or hold our breath. Think of walking into cold water, the first cold swim of the year; we move our breath higher into the chest, and will often even hold our breath. We do the same in the midst of something unpleasant.

This entire region of the body, the thoracic area, is surrounded by 12 ribs. The ribs are the solid foundation that allows the breath to occur and keeps the area safe and protected. The number 12 appears to be a symbolic or "perfect number." There were 12 tribes of Israel, 12 children of Jacob, 12 disciples, and 12 kinds of fruit on Revelation's tree of life.

When looking at imbalance in this central area of the body, it helps to remember the functions of these parts. Our lungs, for example, "let go" minute by minute. When we are required to let go of someone or something before we are ready, we become "broken-hearted"; grief sits heavy on our chest. Many times when I have placed my hands on a client's chest, tears have started to flow. Often the tears turn to sobbing. Deep grief that had been stored in this area of the body could finally be expressed.

The heart and lungs also *receive* the breath of life and are always involved in change and exchange. Sometimes we fear change. We cling to possessions or people, fearing the emptiness of doing without them. Our lungs teach us to let go and receive, in balance, accepting change and knowing there will be an exchange.

The Feet and Legs

The feet are the foundation on which we stand. They support our movement forward. Through our feet we connect with Mother Earth. To stand strong means to feel supported, not just by the ground underneath you but by the people and situations in your life. The left foot and leg may represent our matriarchal lineage, the right our patriarchal lineage.

For some people, understanding their lineage helps them feel strong – they feel they have a firm foundation in life. For others, their heritage may cause them to feel weak and insubstantial. Phrases such as, "I feel like I don't have a leg to stand on," "I feel on shaky ground," or "pulled the rug out from under me," offer clues that something is happening with the foundation of the person. Conversely, "I can stand on my own" affirms our ability to be independent, to stand alone, and to move in the direction we choose.

Various joints make us flexible, able to change direction, to absorb shock, and, at times, to surrender and kneel.

Our legs may also mirror ambivalence, conflict, or fear about the direction we are going or desire to go. We may feel conflict between God calling in one direction, and family expectations pushing us in another. Our support is in question; our muscles may tighten to reflect this emotional, spiritual tension. The left side and right side will usually correspond with the masculine and feminine qualities.

Hips are where we have pockets. Pockets are a place to put away and store things. Where do you put your memories when you don't want to look at them?

In a workshop I attended, I was asked to draw a picture of suffering. I enthusiastically covered a large piece of paper with my images of suffering. When finished, I carefully folded and folded and folded this piece of paper until it was small enough to place in my right hip pocket. At that moment a mental light went on. My right hip is often very painful, with no physical signs of arthritis. This is the place I store much of my emotional and spiritual pain.

Now I know that when I get pain in that hip, I am storing my pain again. It's time to let go of some of it.

The Arms and Hands

We use our arms to express ourselves, to receive with, to care for and to protect ourselves and others. Our hands allow us to work with fine detail, whether creating or receiving. The flexible joints in our arms and our strong muscles let us reach in any direction and carry large or small burdens. We can even use our arms to lift our body, to move ourselves if required.

Disharmony shows up in the arms and shoulders when there is conflict around what to express, when there is a holding back of creativity or a conflict between the heart's desire and duty. It may be a large burden, like "carrying the weight of the world on your shoulders." On the right side, it may reflect a need to express something assertively; the left may have more to do with intuitive, emotional expression.

Our hands are ways we create, we give, and we receive. Touch through our hands is essential in communicating healing qualities. A compassionate loving touch will communicate across all languages.

I remember an elderly Chinese woman in a hospital. She was crying. All attempts to calm her had failed. I simply went up to her, and lovingly touched the center of her chest. She stopped crying instantly, looked at me, and broke into a smile. Her roommate had died that night. Somehow, my communication through touch brought her comfort in her grief.

Our hands are the tools for the love in our hearts. It is no coincidence that "laying on of hands" has been a healing tradition in all faiths and cultures.

The Neck

The neck is situated between the head and the heart. It allows us to turn and see in all directions. It provides a vital passage for the breath of God, for food and nourishment, and for information to reach the rest of the body through the nerves. Through what we see, smell, hear, and taste we determine our safety. The neck determines whether or not we feel safe to breath, to eat, to venture forward.

So we speak of "sticking our neck out" when a situation feels risky, or of "the hair on the back of our neck standing up" when there is danger.

Trauma in the area of the neck is life threatening. So neck problems often reflect our sense of safety. It is also where we express our faith and trust. Despite what we see or hear, we have faith that we will be safe or come through safely.

The neck is also where we call for help. An event in the past such as sexual abuse may still be telling us that life isn't safe.

We stop expression at the neck. Our feelings rise and ask for verbal expression, but we "put a lid on it," sometimes "swallowing our emotions."

So when "dis-ease" settles in the neck area, it is valuable to review what isn't being expressed, what is threatening our safety, or where there is conflict in how we express our heart's (God's) desire or calling.

The Head

The head is "central control" for our human system. We receive input through the sensing of the eyes, the ears, the nose, and the mouth. We use these (as well as touch and intuition) to feed information to the brain, which then transmits decisions and instructions to the body.

Often, emotions will surface to the "top." We then "put a lid on it" or "blow our tops." Or, when we have conflicting information, our "heads" tell us one thing and our "guts" another. We ask, "Does your head rule your heart, or does your heart rule your head?" The head often represents our rational mind; our "gut and our heart" represent another form of wisdom. When body wisdom and head wisdom differ, our bodies will register this. A classic symptom is the headache.

The Upper Abdomen

This is the place where we receive nourishment into the depths of our being, where we digest what is good for us and let go of what we don't need. Our intestinal system has a highly developed process of filtering, discerning, receiving, and releasing.

This is, then, the place we digest our thoughts and experiences, sometimes over and over, to the point where we physically have indigestion or pain. We may take in the feelings of others and feel like we have been "hit in the stomach," or simply feel sick to our stomach. When we swallow our emotions instead of voicing them, we add stress to our digestive system.

The Lower Abdomen

Our bowels are the final filtration system for our intestinal tract. They reabsorb what is valuable from that which is to be released. We then eliminate the waste from our life. If we try to hang on to something toxic, our bowels quickly let us know through pain and bloating that we are out of balance.

So, like the lungs, the bowels teach us what we need to let go of. This may be memories, emotions such as bitterness and rage, or thoughts that are not helpful to our beings. We constantly need to decide what is no longer serving our bodies and beings.

Our entire digestive system reminds us that it is important to decide what nourishes us: physically, emotionally, mentally, and spiritually. Then we can seek the "nutrition" that will promote health on all levels, and be ready to let go of what is not helpful any longer. Life is a process of receiving and letting go, to stay in balance and harmony.

Our Creative Center

To our pelvic area comes the sacred energy of creation. On a physical level – reproduction – we create from this place in our bodies. Here, divine love finds expression and form. A pelvis filled with vital creative life-giving energy allows us to create new life, not only through babies but through our hobbies, our jobs, our gardens.

Unfortunately, this is also the area we often carry the shame of our bodies. Occasionally, this area can "take over," disregarding the wisdom and welfare of the rest of our bodies. It is this area, therefore, that society has often connected with "original sin." Because of fear of sinning, we shut the flow of vital energy down, and live above the waist.

Yet when we feel fully alive, our breath comes deeply into the pelvis, filling our well of life with "living waters."

The Back

The back consists of the pelvis, the spine, and the ribs, with both large and small muscles attached to the bones. These provide a structure to keep us erect, allow us to carry heavy loads on our back, and move and turn with our feet firmly planted. As well, the back provides an intricate channel for our nervous system.

Metaphorically, we put behind us that which we don't want to look at, what we hope is done with, and what we would like to leave behind. We carry loads on our back, both seen and unseen. Phrases such as "spineless" or "carry the cross on our back" are descriptive metaphors for back problems. Here, too, our bodies will mirror betrayal. We use the metaphor, "I've been stabbed in the back," and we talk about "things going on behind our backs." Back symptoms often tell us that all is not well.

The spine is the central core of the back. It consists of 33 bony segments stacked on top of each other. The spine supports the head, provides attachments for the ribs, protection for nerves of the spinal column, and attachment for muscles. Aligning the spine in an erect manner is important in many spiritual practices as a means of allowing God's energy to flow through our bodies with ease.

The Bones

Our bones are the core to which everything else is attached. They are the central foundation from which we derive our form and structure. The prophet Ezekiel recognized this:

> *Thus says the Lord God to these bones:*
> *I will cause breath to enter you, and you shall live,*
> *I will lay sinews on you, and will cause flesh to come upon you,*
> *and cover you with skin, and put breath in you and you shall live.*
> (37:5-6)

From that principle, we might let bones stand for the laws of God, the foundations by which we live and by which the universe functions. When we know the rules, the laws, we feel safe and in right relationship with God.

Symptoms in our bones can often mirror problems at a foundational level. For instance, during a workshop where the group had to discover how to make its own rules and how rules provide necessary structure and form, my bones ached constantly. When I looked deep inside, to dialogue with the aching in my bones, a flood of memories came forth, of times of discomfort when, either as a child or as an adult, in a classroom, a family situation, and even a church community, I had not known the "rules." As an intuitive person, I could usually sense when the "unwritten rules" seemed to conflict with the "written rules." My body was never sure which foundation to rely on.

The Muscles

Most of us recognize the clues our muscles give us when they cry out in pain through strain or spasms. A shoulder massage quickly reveals which spots are tender and sore. Our muscles are necessary for movement, for gesture and expression. They support us and help us eat, breathe, and eliminate.

Any time we respond emotionally, our muscles respond to that feeling. For fear, our muscles prepare us to run away or to fight. With a steady feeling of fear in our lives, our muscles will hold the energy of that emotion; some people have lifelong fear held in the muscles. When you feel anger, where in your body do your muscles tense up? If you resist being pushed to go in a particular direction, where does the tension surface?

Even the tiniest muscle in our body – such as an eye muscle – can tell a story of what has been seen, or perhaps of what we didn't want to see.

We can learn much from the wisdom in our muscles when we are mindful of even the slightest form of tension.

The Blood

Our biblical ancestors thought of blood as the source of life. The absence of blood, like the absence of breath, clearly identified death. So Hebrew sacrifices required life-blood, symbolizing the dedication of a life to God.

Our blood receives the breath of God as life-giving force. Then it flows through the heart, receiving love. It is circulated to each cell in the body, each member of the whole. Finally, it carries the waste products to be cleansed and cleared from the body. Our blood is a communication system, by which hormones and enzymes are transported like little couriers on a highway. It needs to be kept at a balanced pressure, enough pressure to ensure that all parts are nourished, but not so high as to risk a rupture and flood. The blood can not function separate from the whole. It is the essential unifying part, always working to keep the parts nourished, balanced, and in harmony.

When we take the wine, the symbolic "blood of Christ" in Holy Communion, we are receiving the unifying, healing light and love that was sent to restore wholeness and harmony to all "parts" of the world.

Many Ways of Expressing Wisdom

While our bodies will cry out through symptoms and we need to learn to listen to those symptoms, the meaning of each experience is personal. Only the person who has the experience can interpret the actual meaning. A "healer" can only help to focus the listening, to help the person seeking healing identify and interpret the body's wisdom. What is important is that we learn to listen to the wisdom of our bodies, to recognize that our souls speak to us through our bodies and that our bodies do pray for wholeness and harmony.

We need to remember, too, not to leap to conclusions. My aching hip could reveal symptoms of bones and structure, of pockets and storage, of muscles and being held back, or of my right or masculine elements. It takes patience and discernment to unravel the often tangled and overlapped threads of meaning in any symptom.

But by being mindful, deeply present to the symptom, taking the time to listen, the process will unfold, the story will be told, the insight will come, and the transformation and healing will happen.

Healing is both a privilege and a responsibility.
While it is open to anyone, it should not be entered into lightly.
Rochelle Graham *describes some ways of preparing yourself,*
and of applying healing techniques.

6

A Healing Method

When entering into either the role of healer (the one being the instrument of God's grace) or healee (the one receiving), the divine mystery is experienced in concrete ways. The experience may be common to all participating in the healing session, or it may be unique to each individual. Through the healing experience, people develop a personal relationship with the divine. They often have a particular face of God that speaks to them. For example, some people experience profound light and love, others may feel or see the hands of Jesus, still others may experience qualities best described as "mother."

In reading the stories of Christians throughout history as well as the stories of the New Testament, it is clear that people had profound experiences of the divine that were unique and life changing. The words God, Christ and Holy Spirit may have particular faces depending on your experience and your theological understanding.

The Personal Experience of the Trinity

I have found that people's understanding of Christ or of the Holy Spirit is as varied as the people themselves.

In an attempt to understand how that affects the healing that takes place, I did an experiment with several different groups of healers. These people had taken several workshops within the church and were familiar with the basics involved in healing work.

In each exercise, the healer placed his or her hands on the shoulders of the healee. In the first exercise, they invited *God's* energy from the earth to flow through the healer to the healee. After two minutes, both the healer and healee debriefed the exercise and described the experience. The same process was then followed by next asking *Christ* to work through the healer. Following that debriefing, the exercise was repeated a third time focusing on the *Holy Spirit.* Finally, it was done with the *Trinity* combined. The purpose was to discern the variations in what many people experience or name as different aspects, qualities, or faces of God.

What surprised all of us, totaling about 40 people, was that the experience of each aspect of the Trinity was profoundly different. Even more surprising, the experience of individuals in the group was consistently similar.

There were a number of clergy in the group. All who experienced this were in awe of the mystery present during this experiment. The beliefs of the individuals participating did not seem to affect the outcome.

Marcus Borg, Hundere Distinguished Professor of Religion and Culture at Oregon State University and author of *Meeting Jesus Again for the First Time* and *The God We Never Knew*, described, in a lecture I attended, the development of the Trinitarian formula in the fourth century as a means of describing the different faces or masks of God. The word "persons" used in the Nicene Creed meant *persona* or mask. You may find that there is a particular *persona* of God that you feel most comfortable using and which supports your personal relationship with the Divine Mystery.

Preparing Yourself for Healing

When doing healing work, we need to spend time preparing all aspects of our being. Our ability to be an instrument of healing depends on many factors. Self-healing and self-care become an essential focus. A tree needs to be well nourished with roots deep in the earth, it needs a good water supply, unpolluted air, and plenty of light to be strong, grow healthy, and weather the storms. So do we, also, need to be diligent about how we care for all aspects of our self. As authors of this book, each of the three of us has a personal way of preparing. Your particular method will depend on where you are working, who you are working with, and the amount of time you have to prepare.

Both Flora and I do a lot of our work with clients in a room set aside for healing. We usually go into the space to pray and to ask that the space be turned over to the living Christ through the Holy Spirit. We use centering prayer and meditation to bring ourselves to a peaceful quiet place where we feel present to God. We then begin to pray for the person before he or she has even arrived. So essentially the preparation begins well in advance. Of course prior to this, we have also done what self-care is required to ensure our physical needs are looked after.

Wayne has similar ways of preparing himself in his office or car before ministering to people.

Personal Preparation

The body needs to be kept healthy through a well-balanced diet, through drinking lots of water, and through regular exercise, rest, and recreation. Although the energy for healing does not come from one's own bioenergy field, the metabolic energy required to do healing work is usually high. This requires regular eating of high quality, nutritious food. Exercise keeps the body in good shape, and it also helps to keep the lines of energy flow (the acupuncture meridians) open and balanced. Mindful exercise, being aware of your body sensations during activity, also helps to keep the person in the present moment.

Breathing exercises are another way of preparing to do healing work. Yoga and T'ai Chi/Qi Gong are wonderful examples of using movement and breath to fill the body with vital energy and to balance the bioenergy field.

Prior to working with someone, you need to be aware of any emotions of your own. For example, if you have just come from a conflict and are still feeling very angry, this will affect your ability to be a peaceful presence during the healing. You will need to spend time bringing your own emotions back into balance and harmony. This doesn't mean you bury the problem – you either release it into God's hands or set it aside to be dealt with later so that your focus can be clear and peaceful. The goal is to feel more like a peaceful calm lake rather than a stormy sea.

What thoughts are present for you? Is something demanding your attention enough to make it difficult for you to stay fully present with the people you will be working with? You will need to set that situation aside, pray about it, and ensure that it is not present while doing healing work. An example of this is the prayer of confession – letting go, offering up to God that which limits our ability to be an instrument of healing. I call this "making room for more of God's grace and healing light and love."

Being fully present with another person during a healing session is similar to using a magnifying glass. The light pouring through a magnifying glass is focused and therefore more effective and useful. If divine energy is trying to pour through you but your thoughts are focused elsewhere, it diffuses the energy.

Applying Christian Healing

Laying on of hands is using your hands as the instrument of healing, a form of body prayer. In chapter 3, Flora has described how the laying on of hands has been an element of healing in almost all cultures and civilizations in history. The particular method I practice intentionally works within the framework of Christian teachings from scripture and church tradition.

The following instructions do not include healing prayer and anointing, which are described in other chapters.

Prepare the Person Receiving

Make sure that you have permission to work with each person before you begin. Always check if they are comfortable being touched. Also give them permission to give you feedback at any time.

If this is the first time someone is experiencing this form of healing work, take time to explain what you will be doing. I usually use language similar to this: "Are you comfortable being touched? If at any point you aren't comfortable, with my touch, the pressure of my touch, or what you are experiencing, please give me that feedback. I may be actually touching you, or I may be working in your personal space so that you won't feel any direct touch. Now, I am going to take a moment to quietly pray and ask God to work through me and guide my hands. I may ask you questions during this time. Are you comfortable with that?"

If the person I'm working with says "No," I respect that. I'll work quietly within her or his boundaries. I may clarify whether their "No" means they just need a peaceful time, or whether they would experience my questions as invading their privacy.

Center Yourself Again

While your preparation will usually have occurred before the healing session begins, it may be necessary to take a few more moments to prepare.

This is called centering. It requires you to become fully present with the person who is the focus of this session. It means clearing yourself of any distracting thoughts, feelings, and external noises. This requires ongoing discipline.

You may need to bring yourself back to center many times initially. Taking several deep breaths, to breathe in the breath of God, can assist you to connect to the divine central core within yourself. This is the spiritual heart center referred to in scripture. This internal place is connected to God and is an endless fountain of life. It is the place where God's love and compassion can flow through freely.

Being centered means feeling peaceful, aware that your breath is deep and even, you are grounded in your body, connected to a higher source of power. Henri Nouwen in his book *Here and Now* speaks about God's heart being greater than the human heart. He says,

> *The Holy Spirit of God is given to us so that we can become*
> *participants in God's compassion and so*
> *reach out to all people at all times with God's heart.*

Define Your Intention

Once you feel centered – and this may only take a few minutes – it is important to be clear about what you are doing, who is the source of the power, and what you are asking for. This may be a single sentence, or it may be a lengthy prayer. Another way to describe this is stating your intention. It is also a time of aligning with God's will. You may also ask the person receiving what their intention is. This helps to clarify for both the healer and the receiver what is being asked for. I usually use one of these two prayers:

> *May I be an instrument of healing according to divine will*
> *for the highest good of* (name).

> Or

> *Loving healing God, may I be a channel for your healing energy;*
> *allow all that is required to assist* (name) *in her/his healing to*
> *flow through me. Make me a channel of the love and wisdom*
> *of Christ by the power of the Holy Spirit. May I listen with*
> *your ears, may your wisdom guide my words and reveal to*
> *me that which I need to see. We ask for this healing in Christ's*
> *name and according to your will. Amen.*

Avoid mixed intentions. Sometimes we think we're clear in our intention, when our motivation actually differs slightly. You may run into this when working with a close friend or relative; your need to have the other person get better may conflict with their need to be sick.

For example, a woman named Fran described a situation where her husband was sick and unable to go to her family reunion. This created conflict between them. Her need was to have him well and with her at the reunion; his need was to rest and recover in peace, not likely to occur if he went to the reunion. Aligning to God's will in such a situation may mean examining why you are offering the healing session, and who is benefiting from the treatment.

Decide What To Do

The term for gathering information is assessment. A simple explanation is to gather enough information to know what to ask for in your prayers of intention, to have some idea where to start. Assessment begins with the first contact. It may be verbal, visual, or aural; it may come through intuition; it may come as physical sensation in your hands.

There are many sources of information and many methods of gathering it. Assessment may involve an in-depth analysis, or a brief asking of what is needed. The depth of assessment will depend on whether you have training in interviewing and clinical assessment, as in nursing or counseling. But any perceptive lay person or clergy can gather much useful information:

1. **Listen**. Listen to the greeting, the phrases used to describe what is happening. Often there will be a metaphor: "I feel like the rug has been pulled out from under me," or "This is breaking my heart." Such phrases offer a clue to what the body is communicating. Listen for both the quality of the voice as well as the actual words. Is the voice strong or does it sound fragile? What is the reason for coming? Keep in mind that it will often take several visits before the person feels safe enough to reveal real needs. When the safe place is created, the person will share more deeply. By listening to the wisdom in their words, you'll know the problem. Our job is to listen to both the literal and symbolic clues.

2. **Observe**. Note the facial expressions, the body positions, the walk. Are the shoulders up near the ears? Is the face grimacing? Does the body appear relaxed, or tense and tight? Is there a bright smile while telling a sad story? Is the breathing shallow or deep? Paying careful attention to seemingly small physical details will reveal much about the person. Some healers are able to see more than the physical body, such as the bioenergy field or aura. The aura may look like a soft light several inches from the person or appear as colors. Others might simply perceive the brightness of the face, noticing a contrast in light or dullness.

Use Your Hands to Gather Information

Now you have some clues where to use your hands to give you further information. The bioenergy field can extend several feet out from the body. Most of us sense this when someone stands too close to us. We back up because they have entered our space. This is space we claim even though it isn't a visible space.

In this way, your hands can feel what is happening off the person's body.

This is often difficult for new healers. They don't feel confident with it. It requires developing a heightened sensitivity in the nerve endings of the palm and fingers. For some, this may take considerable time to develop. It is similar to developing the skill of reading Braille. At first, when reading Braille, you feel only bumps; later, Braille becomes a readable language. In the same way, you can develop sensitivity to "reading" the energy around the body.

But whether or not you are able to feel much with your hands will not limit your ability to be an effective instrument of divine healing. I was fortunate, because I could feel things immediately, and I've found that my sensitivity has continued to increase. My husband, on the other hand, has taken several years to develop this skill. Yet I have received many wonderful treatments from him during that time.

A way of "waking up" your hands, of helping to draw attention to the sensations in them, is to rub your palms together vigorously for 30 seconds. This increases the circulation in the hands, and focuses your awareness fully on your hands.

To feel the bioenergy field through the use of your hands begin moving your hands softly through the space around the person's body. Simply be aware of any sensations in your palms. Your hands are in receptive mode; you are not doing a treatment at this point.

Now begin on the front of the body, two to four inches from the body. Start at the head and slowly work your way down the body to the feet. If the person is sitting, you can also assess the back and each side. At this point simply notice whether the bioenergy field feels the same over the entire body, making note of any differences. You may experience temperature sensations, tingling, density, or pressure. These are all qualities that our nerve endings can register. Since health consists of wholeness, balance, and harmony, your hand scan assesses differences in balance and wholeness.

Once you have done a scan close to the body, you can repeat it at 6–10 inches, 12–20 inches, and even farther out, at a distance of several feet. As your hands become more sensitive you will perceive distinct layers. This scan is similar to checking the layers or rings of a tree. Each layer differs, depending on whether it relates to a physical, emotional, or mental problem, or whether it affects a person's entire being – including their spirit. How much the problem or suffering affects the person will be mirrored in the bioenergy field.

Trust Your Intuitions

Some people gather their information intuitively. Often this is described as knowing in your gut. Proverbs 2:2, 10 speak of wisdom coming into your heart when you incline your heart toward God, and 1 Corinthians 12 describes the gifts of the Holy Spirit. In gathering information that you may be unsure about, pray for clarity, pray that the information be revealed only as you need it, and pray only for the highest good of the person involved. This respects boundaries of privacy, and ensures that only what is required is revealed.

I recall working on a man dying of cancer in the hospital. I was helping him to relax. He was very agitated and somewhat confused. As he started to settle down, I heard a voice say to me, "Ask him if he wants a beer." It was Sunday morning in the hospital; I was not going to heed this voice. But the voice got louder and quite insistent. Still I ignored it, fearing embarrassment at saying this with the family around.

Finally the words came out of my mouth. The man sat up and said, "You would do this for me?" His family asked if that is what he wanted. He replied quite strongly that this was important to him.

I finished the treatment and went home, knowing that this man would die soon. His family called later to say that they had gone out and bought the beer, and brought his favorite stein from home. He was German; he had not been able to drink his beloved beer for more than a year. They described a wonderful final celebration where they all shared beer together. The man became very lucid. He sat up drinking his beer from the stein. Before this he had only been able to have liquids spooned into his mouth. Shortly after, he died.

If I had continued to ignore the voice, that family would not have had this quality of goodbye.

Work with the Energy

A basic premise of treatment is that the life force or healing energy of God moves to fill us. For the filling to occur, we may need to let go, to make space. Just as our food, water, and breath move through us, so does this vital life force.

So treatment aims at either helping to clear and spread areas where these vital forces are thick or piled up, or helping to fill thin places, or a combination of the two.

This is a very simple way to look at treatment. There may be times when our hands will be moved to where the mystery of God's Holy Spirit is particularly acting. Paul's prayer from Ephesians 3:18-19 fits here:

I pray that you may have the power…to know the love of Christ
that surpasses knowledge, so that you may be filled with all the
fullness of God.

There are times when the healer is filled with all the fullness of God and the experience will surpass knowledge.

Whether you are actively moving your hands or not, remember that any time you reach out to touch another person, or an animal, or even a plant in a loving and compassionate manner, you have been an instrument for healing. Being a vessel for God's healing power means that the energy and resources do not come from ourselves but through us. This is the importance of centering and of setting intention.

Research scientist Janet Quinn demonstrated in her early work in the 1970s that persons going through exactly the same motions as healers, but without the intention to help or heal (they were counting backwards instead), produced no measurable benefit. The patients of nurses who clearly intended to heal showed significant reductions in anxiety levels; the patients of nurses who were simply going through the motions did not.

Learn the Right Techniques

Why do you need to learn technique? When learning something for the first time, you often need to spend time in skill development and practice. The source of healing energy is from God and is a gift of the spirit, but we have to train our hands, eyes, heart, and physical body to handle this new gift. Most people feel more confident when they have a set of instructions to guide them first. When they are comfortable with the basics, they are more able to let the gift of the spirit take form. When learning to cook or bake you follow a recipe until you are confident in what it takes to be successful. Then you can allow the creative spirit to take over. The same is true for healing.

Certain skills are required to work successfully with the bioenergy field. The basics are given here, and you will find other techniques in Appendix B.

Essentially there are two ways to use your hands. You may move them, or keep them still. And you can do it on or off the body.

As you become more skilled in allowing yourself to be guided by the Holy Spirit, your hands will be shown what to do. Until then here are some basic guidelines.

1. Begin with your hands off the body. Reaching above the head, move from top to bottom, from center to the edges. This is a bit like following the branches of an evergreen tree as they grow from the top down to the base at the ground.

2. Make sure that you are working from the head all the way to the feet.

3. Use very slow and gentle movements. This is to help the flow of life force to move through the body and to clear any resistance to this movement. It's like slowly moving your hands through water, helping to clear any debris or mud that may be clogging a stream.

4. You may notice an area that is not clearing well. Even though you move your hands through the bioenergy field, there may still be a sensation of heat, tingling, or congestion that doesn't seem to change easily.

5. Focus on this area with your hands by moving them in this area like an air massage or by moving one hand after the other through the place of focus.

Fill the Energy Voids

At any time during the intervention you may feel called or drawn to place your hands on a particular area. This may be done through direct touch with the person's body, or by placing your hands just above the body.

Leaving your hands in place, invite God's healing energy to flow into your hands. Keep them there until you feel ready to take them off. One clue – they will feel stuck in the same position until it is time to take your hands off. If you are not sure, you may ask, "Would you like my hands left on or are you ready to have them lift off?"

Reassessing the Needs

At any time, you may choose to reassess with your hands, or with a verbal assessment, or through any of the ways described earlier. In reassessing, notice what has changed, what is different from the initial assessment. As you do so, sense whether you need to continue with further intervention or draw the treatment to a close.

Closing a Healing Experience

While receiving a treatment, the receiver may have experiences ranging from deep relaxation, altered consciousness, falling asleep, or even reliving a deep emotional experience. The person will need time to feel fully awake, alert and present before carrying on with normal activities. Here are some suggestions:

1. Hold their feet and gently massage the lower leg towards the foot. This helps them connect to their physical body again, and helps the "grounding" process.

2. Spend some time before they leave, talking about the experience. In group facilitation terms, invite them to "debrief." Asking how their body feels will help them come to the present "now."

3. Pray. It is always appropriate to close with prayers for the continued healing of the person, as well as prayers for anyone else who may be involved in the person's life.

4. Offer a final prayer releasing the person or persons into God's care.

These are the basics of using your hands as an instrument for God's healing energy. As you learn to deepen your connection to God and to Christ through your heart, you will find the Holy Spirit will begin to move your hands, and your trust in this guidance will deepen.

Absent Healing Happens Too

Anytime that you pray for someone, you facilitate healing – even at a distance. That distance may be the neighbor beside you or a friend traveling halfway around the world.

I recall once waking up abruptly in the middle of the night with a dream about a very dear friend traveling in India. In my dream, this person was in trouble, needing help. At that point I began to pray daily for this person, imagining God's light and love surrounding her. I asked that she be helped in whatever manner possible. There was no way to contact this friend, to confirm the message of the dream. But I trusted the strength of the message and knew that in any case my friend would benefit from this prayer.

On her return from India, my friend confirmed the dream. She said that she had specifically reached out to me, trusting that I would get the message and send help. She also confirmed that help had indeed arrived.

If God needs us to facilitate healing, we will be called on to assist even if it is around the world.

Unconsciously, without even consciously thinking about another person, Flora sometimes picks up that person's condition from a distance. She will feel another's distressed condition of mind, heart, or body as her own. She has had to learn to differentiate between what is "hers" and what is not. She has to ask first, "Is this mine?" When it is, then she prays for herself. When it is not, she prays to raise her own energy, by tuning to Christ, so that whoever is tuned in to her may come into resonance with Christ's healing power. Her chapter on prayer speaks about intercessory prayer, prayer without words, and prayer of visualization. All of these can be used for distance healing.

In the same way, your hand movements can influence someone at a distance. You can do the same treatment you would if the person were present, and ask God that the person receive this.

One morning I received a call asking me to work on a man who was bedridden, noncommunicative, and refusing any assistance. He had been that way for at least a week. I asked the family what they wanted me to do. I felt helpless, since he refused to see anyone. They asked for a distance healing session. I agreed to try it.

After quietly centering with prayer, I proceeded to my treatment room. I asked God that this treatment transfer to the man who needed it. I asked that he receive according to God's will and in God's time.

I then proceeded to do the treatment called "The Sacred Chakra Spread" (outlined in Appendix B) just as though the man were present in the room. At the end of the treatment, I offered a prayer of thanks and released the man into God's hands, just as I would if he were there. The next morning the family called to say the man was up, shaved, and eating. I was again in awe of how God works.

In much the same way, Flora and Wayne had rented a retreat house for a group. Ruth was their cook. When they arrived, Ruth was busy making preparations, but was experiencing great pain in her legs. She had no time to stop for a treatment. So with her permission, Flora and Wayne secluded themselves in another room, prepared themselves, and began to perform absent healing on her legs. They visualized her before them. Flora worked in the front and Wayne worked behind her. They could feel the same sensations in their hands as if she were present. When they were done and returned to the kitchen, Ruth told them the pain was gone.

Any of the treatments described in this book can be done at a distance. Of course, it's usually a good idea to have the other person aware of the time of the treatment, in order to be in a relaxed, centered and receptive state – and not at work or involved in an activity such as driving along the highway!

If you are unsure what to do, simply center through prayer and ask God to use your hands, heart, and mind to facilitate healing in the person. I often visualize God's light and love surrounding the person. Later, when I have an opportunity to do in-depth work, I will again center and ask God to reveal through the Holy Spirit what is the matter with the person. Almost always, I will be shown what is wrong, and shown what to do.

But I have to admit that the first time I was called to work on a newborn in extreme distress and on life support systems, I really had no idea what to do. I could not physically make contact with the baby. So I centered and prayed, "God, I have no idea why this is happening, or of what to do. I don't have a sense of the outcome. But please, if in any way you can use me, these are your hands, this is your heart, and I am here open to being your instrument. Please allow me to help this little being in any way possible."

At that point, I felt the presence of the baby. I was aware that this little girl was in deep pain. My hands began to work very fast as though I were pulling the pain out of the baby. This continued for about 15 minutes. Slowly my hands stopped. I was aware that the pain and distress had changed to absolute peace in this little being. The little girl died several days later, after having several wonderful days with her loving parents.

I will never know how much this prayer time helped this little girl and her family. But I believe deeply that whenever I am called upon, God always has a reason.

The biggest impediment to a ministry of healing
may well be rational skepticism about the power of prayer.
Wayne Irwin *felt that doubt, and set out to identify*
the often overlooked scientific evidence
supporting healing through prayer.

7

The Power of Prayer

I was introduced to the ministry of prayer for healing within the church by a colleague, Bill Slinn, a United Church minister serving in Mississauga. Bill held a regular healing service in his church, and shared occasional stories of his experience with me. But Bill was regarded by most of his associates within the presbytery as unconventional; and almost everyone seemed to ignore what he was doing.

I had been trained in the scientific method prior to entering seminary. I constantly questioned Bill about what could be measured. But I was reluctant to introduce a healing ministry into the church I served, Lowville United. In my ministerial training, there had been no mention whatsoever of healing. It did not seem to be considered a part of the United Church culture.

To reintroduce any such ministry into the United Church, I believed, would require an adequate scientific rationale.

In the late 1970s, Bill conducted a series of workshops on the ministry of prayer for healing. I attended. And as I listened to anecdotal testimony of the effect of the laying on of hands from the persons in attendance, I recognized a description in human terms of what physics calls "inductance." Inductance, briefly put, is a relationship between two unconnected electrical circuits. Under certain circumstances, a current flowing in one circuit causes – or "induces" – a current to flow in the second circuit.

Since electric currents are known to flow within the human system, there must be some kind of electromagnetic field surrounding our bodies. Through prayer and meditation, the healer, the person laying on hands, would serve to bring his or her body and electromagnetic field into some semblance of harmony, into a state of divine balance. And when the healer's body was then brought into proximity with the recipient's, there would be a beneficial influence upon that person's system, by induction. A force of some kind would affect the field of the recipient, moving the recipient's system closer to that balance, and thus enhancing healing.

With that limited preliminary understanding, I began my quest into the science of healing prayer.

The Accepted Experimental Method

Science recognizes controlled studies. It investigates specific questions in which the variables have been limited. Limiting the variables is necessary to ensure that the outcome really depends on the particular process or method being tested. For example, using seeds or beans or plants rather than persons as "subjects" of an experiment in intercessory prayer (prayer on behalf of something or someone else, rather than petition for oneself) eliminates the possibility that the outcome could be influenced by suggestion or by the subject's own prayer.

A "control" group is also always needed. For the control group, all conditions are the same, except for the one variable being tested. And so-called "double-blind" studies eliminate even the possibility that the outcome could be influenced by the investigator's thoughts or intention. In a double-blind study, neither the subjects nor the operator know who is in the tested group or the control group; and furthermore, the operator does not know what the study is testing and therefore cannot possibly influence its outcome by anticipating a particular result.

Good scientific methodology has developed as a way of preventing us from deceiving ourselves about the truth of our hunches. For that reason good tests involve large "samples." Experiments involving only a handful of subjects are not considered as statistically significant as those involving hundreds. The Randolph Byrd study of the effect of intercessory prayer on heart patients was greeted with such interest because approximately 400 subjects were involved.

Randolph Byrd, a cardiologist, performed clinical studies at San Francisco General Medical Center from August 1982 through May 1983 on the therapeutic effects of prayer at a distance. He used a randomized double-blind method with coronary care patients to follow the results of 192 patients receiving intercessory prayer from Christian prayer groups across the United States. Another 201 un-prayed-for patients were used as a control group (though it is recognized that others outside the experiment may have prayed for them). Statistically signifi-cant outcomes in a number of areas of investigation showed that the prayed-for patients did better. They required, for example, less frequent ventilatory assis-tance, antibiotics, and diuretics than the control group. Prayer at a distance made the difference!

Byrd's is not the only large-scale experiment demonstrating the effects of prayer. Dr. Seán Ó'Laoire, a Roman Catholic priest in San Francisco, described *An Experimental Study of the Effects of Intercessory Prayer-at-a-distance on Self-Esteem, Anxiety and Depression,* as his Ph.D. thesis (Palo Alto, Institute of Transpersonal Psychology, May 1993). The controlled, randomized, double-blind study used 90 "agents" or people who would pray; 259 who would be prayed for; and a control group of 147. The agents were given photos of their subjects, and kept individual prayer journals. They prayed for their subjects for a least 15 minutes each day. Five standard psychological tests were adminis-tered to the 496 participants, before and after a 12-week period of prayer. The results demonstrated the prayed-for groups' statistically "significant improve-ment" in self-esteem, anxiety states and traits, depression, and mood disorders in general, compared to the control group.

Those who did the praying also improved in their psychological health over the test period – and at a rate significantly greater than that of the prayed-for subjects!

If there were just one or two studies of the beneficial effect of loving inten-tion and prayer upon the health and well-being of a group of subjects, we might well treat it with skepticism and caution. However, there are over 150 pub-lished reports of controlled studies of such healing work, of which more than half meet all the criteria to be significant.

A Worthy Complement

It seems pointless to further question whether healing works. It does – period! The questions that now need to be addressed are *how* it works, and how we can attune ourselves to receive or achieve the greatest benefit for all.

Daniel J. Benor, an American psychiatrist, has been gathering information about such healing studies for many years. In his multiple volume work, *Heal-ing Research*, he offers reviews and critiques of these studies. By identifying the strengths and weaknesses of each, he forwards the view that "bioenergy medicine" or "healing work" is a worthy complement to conventional medicine. Herbert Benson, the Harvard medical doctor, lecturer, researcher, and author of *The Relaxation Response* and *Timeless Healing*, likens this "healing work" to one of the three legs on a milking stool. The other two are the patient's own active and informed participation, and conventional or "allopathic" medicine. We need all three – or the stool falls over!

Some of us within the church need no scientific rationale. In fact, for some the search for scientific explanation is an affront to their faith. But for those who may have lost their faith, who have never developed it, who need encouragement, or who would simply like to know, there is so much evidence that to doubt the efficacy of prayer is to betray one's ignorance of the facts.

Effect on Bacteria and Fungus Culture

One of the simplest experiments demonstrates that intentional healing prayer can retard the growth of bacteria and fungus.

There have been many reports of one person's prayer accelerating another's recuperation from chronic infection. Presumably, this intentional healing work inhibits bacterial growth, but only as a complement to conventional antibiotic therapy, not as a replacement.

Beverly Rubik, Director of the Center for Frontier Sciences of Temple University in Philadelphia, conducted a study in the 1970s with renowned healer Olga Worrall. Olga was invited to lay hands on three groups of salmonella bacteria – normal, chemically inhibited, or nutritionally starved – in carefully controlled tests of her known ability to influence growth. Even though the experiments were conducted according to "double-blind" standards, in that Olga did not know what the procedure was testing, she was able to remotely ascertain information about the status of the bacterial targets. Though this was not a part of the experiment, it indicated that information flowed both ways between the healer and the subject.

The Benefit of Blessing

The biblical Acts of the Apostles (19:12) claims that healing could be conveyed by handkerchiefs and aprons. This has been put to the test with plants and animals, using water and cotton wool. The laying on of hands, with the mental loving intention to heal, upon a flask of water, which is then poured upon plants, has been shown to provide the same measurable benefit as the direct laying on of hands. The same holds for similar action upon cotton wool which is then fastened to an animal's wound.

This suggests that there is an actual benefit from prayer over an antibiotic or over the water in which it is to be dissolved. Medicine that has been blessed can be a later blessing to the patient.

This kind of evidence challenges the attitude of a minister I worked with many years ago. He did not believe in the value of prayed blessings. Privately, for example, he scorned "saying grace" over the food we eat. He would "ask the blessing" in public only because it was his job, but would never do it in his own home. Given the accumulated evidence today, that minister would be hard-pressed to sustain his skepticism.

The Spindrift Saga

In the 1970s a small group of Christian Scientists began a project to translate into experimentally verifiable terms the teachings of their founder, Mary Baker Eddy, about the scientific validity of prayer. The group was severely reproached for doing so. Although Mrs. Eddy had asserted that demonstration had a place within the church alongside reason and revelation, the church she founded now took a stand against these experimental tests. Any use of mental power, not strictly classified as prayer, was classified as "psychic," and thus, by definition, was unworthy of attention by serious Christians.

Fortunately, their church's disapproval did not curtail the work of this investigative group. Nor did the group's members, at any point, compromise their commitment to Christ. They continued in the spirit of Eddy, in obedience to their own sense of the divine will for their work. Their studies came to be known as "The Spindrift Experiments." Their findings were astounding, although every day these experimenters had to carry the cross of the intellectual and emotional disapproval of their faith community. Within the Christian Science establishment, the Spindrift reports were classified as "heresy."

Since we're discussing definitions, it is perhaps worth noting that heresy is not the teaching of something untrue. Rather, it is the overemphasis of something true, to the detriment of some other aspect of truth. For example, teaching the humanity of Jesus is not heretical, unless it ignores his divinity. The emphasis on an intellectual understanding of one's Christian faith is not heretical, unless it ignores the importance of the development of the personal inner life in relationship with Jesus.

It appears, in other words, that "heresy" – which has always been present somewhere within the religious scene – has a place in God's grand scheme of things. It has something to do with stimulating growth into wisdom. A Muslim adage says,

> *Unless I have been charged with heresy a thousand times,*
> *I have not yet spoken the truth.*

Three Significant Factors

The Spindrift group initially designed experiments simply to show that prayer works. But in so doing, they consistently found three significant factors:

- There had to be a "loving intelligence" involved.
- Stress made a difference.
- So did the amount of prayer offered.

They first placed some rye grass seeds in vermiculite, divided them into two equal groups, and laid a string across the container to mark the division. Then they prayed for the plants on one side of the string, and not for the others. At the end of the test, there were significantly more rye grass shoots in the prayed-for section than in the other – yet all that divided them was a string.

This was their first indication that something about the effect of prayer could be measured.

They then placed their seeds under some stress by putting salt into the water they used to keep the vermiculite moist. They repeated this test several times, with differing amounts of salt. Each time they prayed for plants on one side of a dividing string. They discovered that the measurable effect was greater when the subjects were under stress. The more stress, the greater the measurable effect.

Next, they asked: "Does it matter how much we pray? If someone prays for 10 minutes, and someone else prays for 20 minutes, is it the same amount of prayer? Or is it doubled?"

To test their question, they put together four boxes containing soy beans. One they marked "Control." The other three, they marked as "X," "Y," and "Z." All the beans were weighed and watered daily. The X, Y, and Z beans were also prayed for daily. First they prayed for the X and Y beans, together. Then they prayed for the Y and Z beans, together. Thus the Y beans received twice as much prayer as the X and Z beans. The increase in the growth of the Y beans, compared with the control beans, in each test, was always approximately equal to the sum of the amounts that the X and Z beans increased.

In other words, twice as much prayer had twice as much effect.

Identity Field Theory

The Spindrift group did other experiments, which suggest that plants act according to some overarching principle! They placed plants in enriched soil that would accelerate their growth, and other plants in soil so polluted that it would inhibit the growth. They prayed for all of the plants as a unit, asking simply that they be moved toward their divinely intended identity. The first plants slowed their growth, while the others quickened their growth.

That surprising result led to a new question: "What is the 'source' of the information that informs each plant how to behave?"

They took soy beans, then, and soaked them. Some they oversoaked. Others they undersoaked. Then they prayed for all the beans as a unit, comparing them with a control group of other soy beans for which they did not pray. The oversoaked beans released some of their water. The undersoaked beans retained more of their water than the control.

Then they let the beans dry out. As drying continued, even the oversoaked beans that had been releasing more water than the control group now began to retain more water than the control group beans.

So when the need was to release water, the healing prayer helped them do it. When the need was to retain water, the healing prayer helped them to do that. Healing prayer, they observed, is answered according to need.

That led to a another question: "How does the prayer know which seeds to help?" and "How does the prayer know which way to help them?"

Their conclusions became what is now known as "Identity Field Theory" – a concept paralleled in some ancient esoteric teachings of the Eastern sciences, and echoed in the contemporary morphogenic theories of biologist Rupert Sheldrake. The theory proposes that in prayer we are in direct contact with the Universal Mind – for Christians, with the Loving Intelligence of God. In making a heart link with the entity for which we pray, we add focus and additional energy to what this Intelligence is already endeavoring to provide – the needed information to move the entity towards its divinely intended destiny.

Robert Owen published the findings of the Spindrift group in his book, *Qualitative Research: The Early Years.* For our purposes in this book, here is a summary of findings related to our ministry of "healing from the heart."

The Bridge for Prayer

It appears that an "associational link," or a "heart connection," is the bridge across which prayer power flows. Such a link does not appear to exist in either space or time.

This Spindrift conclusion coincides with current examination of the interface between the dimension of space/time and the realm of dreams and archetypes – the "dimension of knowledge" – reported by William Gough and Robert Shacklett in California, and published in *Subtle Energies*. Their work is based upon the conceptual theories of mathematician Roger Penrose, in Cambridge, England. Penrose published his speculations in *The Emperor's New Mind* and *Shadows of the Mind*. His focus is "twistor space" – what things look like at "the Planck length," 10^{-32} centimeters (a decimal point followed by 32 zeros, with a 1 in the 33rd decimal place). Such a dimension is as small in comparison to an atom as an atom is to an ordinary pea. Penrose shows that, at such unimaginably small sizes, both distance and time are meaningless, and that the movement of information, from one dimension to another, does not involve either space or time.

It also seems that this heart link is more an element of consciousness rather than of material energy or of its bound form – matter.

However, as might be surmised, the Spindrift testing indicates that when any affinity or associational link is weakened, the effectiveness of prayer diminishes. This supports the view that "the loving of the other" is the first step in praying for the well-being of that person or thing.

Sometimes this loving intentional thought seems to have unexpected or unintended effects. Entrenched personal thought patterns may interfere, for example. Other heart connections may intrude, even unconsciously.

The effectiveness of the healing prayer also appears to have a direct relationship to the strength of the heart connection. The more clearly the one who is praying is aware of what or who is being prayed for, the greater the apparent effect of the prayer. For our prayers to have measurable effect, it seems that we need to have a clear conceptual awareness of our "target." The experimental results also suggest that persistence – keeping at it – tends to intensify and strengthen the heart connection.

A Definable Target

The Spindrift experimenters did not have to pray for individual seeds. It seems there is no loss of prayer effect, as long as the one praying can conceptualize all the individuals in a group as some sort of unit. That is, say, all the seeds in area X or Y. What does not work, however, is a vague generalization – such as "everyone in the world who is grieving."

The crucial element seems to be a conceptual whole in the mind of the healer. Thus, one can pray for a person, or for a family, or for a community, or for a nation, with no dividing up of the effect. When certain American cities were prayed for a few years ago, their reported crime rates dropped. This finding would support the validity of such a practice.

Identity-directed Prayer

Prayer also seems to work best when it is directed to the divine view of what is normal and right for that person or entity. Such prayer is not tainted by human desire. It doesn't ask tomato plants to grow just so that I can get more tomatoes!

This kind of prayer can be called "identity-directed." Its intent is always to return the body to the optimum condition for its normal functioning, according to God's point of view, without presuming what that will be. Asking for "God's highest good" is always appropriate, without needing to lay out particulars.

It seems that identity-directed prayer continually moves the subjects toward their personal norms, toward those states of form and function which are individually best for them. As difficult as it may be to think of "force" as being somehow intelligent, loving, decisive, and aware of needs, in each test which the Spindrift group performed, the prayer appeared to somehow link the subject to some kind of loving intelligence that informed the subject how to move toward its own norms.

The Intelligence Differentiates Beneficially

Identity-directed prayer appears to enhance the development of every entity it touches. Whatever it is directed towards is clearly "blessed." This loving intelligence does not discriminate, and it does not compete. Whatever is prayed for receives what is best for it, in relation to its environment.

This is a central finding in every experimental test the Spindrift group carried out with "identity-directed" prayer. When prayer was for seeds or beans or yeast or mold, in different conditions – the same prayer at the same time – the loving intelligence somehow determined what was best for each individual entity. The direction of the effect – to encourage or retard growth, to increase or decrease water retention, for example – varied with each entity, according to its individual need.

To accomplish this, the power of prayer sometimes had caused change in some very complicated and sophisticated ways involving internal chemistry and electrical balance – things that those doing the praying knew nothing about. Obviously, they did not need to know.

Prayer Identifying with God's Thought

The name chosen for the Spindrift work – "Qualitative Research" – arises from the awareness that there appear to be two strains of consciousness that underlie the nature of the world. One is *quantitative*, the other *qualitative*. Scientists, and most of humanity, consider power to be a quantitative entity; it can be weighed and measured. On the other hand, theologians and persons considering reality on the spiritual plane understand power also to be qualitative, an actuality of divine goodness, of love and merciful judgment.

"Qualitative thought," then, is prayer identified with the thought of God, prayer that always heals. Non-qualitative thought (or negative qualitative thought) would be prayer sullied by human emotion, human will, and the desire to control. This negative kind of qualitative thought is nevertheless certainly powerful enough to cause effects, but it is connected to human goals and objectives, rather than to divine ones. It does not always heal, nor does it always move things in the direction of God's will. But it can move things.

Our petitions that ask for "God's highest good" are examples of qualitative thought. Prayers that expect God to carry out our personal goals and objectives, with specific instructions requesting the kind of outcome we want, are examples of the other.

This distinction gives us an insight into the demonic element of some forms of faith healing, the use of suggestion to manipulate another, and the imaging of desired outcomes in its various forms. All of these push results in the direction of the will of the healer(s). But such actions have no inherent, built-in reference to the divine will.

We Are to Have Faith In the Loving Intelligence

Faith healing and other forms of prayer directed toward human goals are certainly powerful. Like the placebo effect in medication, they work best when the mind is engaged, emotions aroused, will strengthened, and faith intensified. When all these elements are linked to particular circumstances, and when the specified goal direction happens to coincide with the divine view of the need at hand, healing – even curing, in some instances – seems to occur.

But if the two do not coincide, the hoped-for effect may not happen. The prayer may seem to go unanswered, because the human intention may be working at cross-purposes with the divine intention. The universal loving intelligence always desires to move the subject towards its particular destiny – which may not be the same as the hopes and the wishes of its family, friends and neighbors.

Some people are comfortable using their bodies in a ministry of healing, some are not. Fortunately, there exists an honorable tradition of healing that requires only a connection of the heart. It's called prayer, and Flora Litt explores the various kinds of prayer we practice.

8

Ways of Praying

There are probably as many definitions of prayer as there are readers of this book.

We are familiar with some forms of prayer in the church: praise, confession, assurance, thanksgiving, petition, supplication (prayer for ourselves), and intercession (prayer for others). But prayer is more than any one form or activity.

What Is Prayer Itself?

Ron DelBene, Episcopal priest and spiritual director, has made this wonderfully concise statement:

> *Many of us believe it is up to us to pray in a way that reaches God.*
> *I believe we are in the presence of God at all times,*
> *and prayer is being attentive to that presence.*

We are like fish in the sea. We swim in a sea of interconnected energy which we do not see. We take it for granted. Catherine of Siena says,

> *The soul is in God and God in the soul,*
> *just as the fish is in the sea and the sea in the fish.*

We live and move and have our being in God. Our prayer can be understood as awareness of living in the presence, the love, and the power of God.

Yet many of us have persistent doubts and questions concerning prayer. To pray for ourselves or to enter into prayer ministry for another, we need to turn toward these doubts and questions, not away from them. God will give us the understanding and faith we need to be confident in prayer.

The Reason We Pray

Does God really hear us when we pray? This is the first step of faith. God always hears our prayer, whether shouted, whispered, groaned, or silently breathed. God perceives the yearnings of our hearts, as well as the thoughts of our minds and the words of our lips. For God who is ever-present with us, knows us through and through.

If God knows our need before we ask, then why pray? Because we can't help it! We may as well admit it. There is an instinctive longing, a reaching toward One already known somewhere deep within the soul. Our heart aches spiritually – and perhaps physically – until we acknowledge the relationship with God in which we already exist. We have a knowing so deep within us that we have to work hard to deny it! Sadly, some people do deny it.

I sometimes wonder if much profanity, "taking the Lord's name in vain," is actually prayer. Could this frustration and anger betray an unexpressed yearning for relationship with God?

We pray because we instinctively know from whom we have come. A story tells of a preschooler begging his mother to let him have some time alone with the newborn baby in their home. The mother hesitates. But because of the child's persistence, she finally agrees to let him have a few moments alone with the baby. She has a baby monitor on in the baby's room, and she listens carefully. She hears the older child enter the room and approach the crib. After a moment of silence, she hears her little boy softly say, "Tell me about God. I'm beginning to forget."

Wordsworth, in *Intimations of Immortality*, penned these beautiful words:

> *Our birth is but a sleep and a forgetting...*
> *Not in entire forgetfulness,*
> *And not in utter nakedness,*
> *But trailing clouds of glory do we come*
> *From God, who is our home.*

All of us came into this world "trailing clouds of glory." We came knowing who God is, and knowing ourselves as spiritual beings. Life in this dimension can cause our certainty to become clouded. We can become forgetful. Yet there is within us a spiritual instinct that can lead us to remembering, if we desire it and allow it to happen. In the center of our being, in our heart center, we can get in touch with our knowing once more.

We have all been touched by Love, for Love is with us in this world. God is with us; we are not alone. We believe it, and so we pray; we open ourselves up to Love.

It has been said that prayer changes things. But nothing changes more than the one who prays.

If, in our prayer, we put faith-filled attention on what we believe God is able and willing to do, the energies of our whole being begin to resonate with the spiritual energy of the Christ. If our prayers are in accord with the high and loving purposes of God, miraculous things can come to be.

Flexing Our Prayer Muscles

As humans, perhaps our greatest temptation is to make God in our own image. That makes our God too small, too limited, too capricious to be trusted to attend to our great need!

Scripture speaks to our unbelief. In the words of the angel to Jesus' mother Mary,

> *For nothing will be impossible with God.* (Luke 1: 37)

This faith statement is echoed by Jesus himself to his disciples:

> *For mortals it is impossible, but for God all things are possible.*
> (Matthew 19:26)

Jesus assured us that God is willing to heal. But we do not do this by bargaining, by trying to ingratiate ourselves with God. Rather, we take a step in prayer, and learn from God's response. We do not learn to walk until we have learned to stand. We do not try to pray for the rebuilding of a heart valve until we have practiced praying for a headache. So we pray as we are able. And our ability increases as we flex our prayer muscles.

The Intention of the Heart

In an old Hasidic tale, a poor farmer was on his way back from market when the wheel of his wagon came off in the middle of the woods. Stranded, he discovered he did not have his prayer book with him. It distressed him that this day should pass without saying his prayers.

So he made up this prayer: "I have done something very foolish, Lord. I came away from home this morning without my prayer book, and my memory is so bad that I cannot recite a single prayer without it. So here is what I am going to do: I shall recite the alphabet five times very slowly, and you, to whom all prayers are known, can put the letters together to form the prayers I can't remember."

And the Lord said to his angels, "Of all the prayers I have heard today, this one was without doubt the best, because it came from a heart that was simple and sincere."

We do not necessarily need words to pray. Adam Clarke writes, "Prayer requires more of the heart than the tongue." It is not the fine words we may say, or the quantity of them, but what is in our heart that counts with God. St. John of the Cross, affirms this in his teaching: "The language that God hears best is the silent language of love." Sometimes we have only silence with which to pray.

Yet we humans most commonly communicate in words. Or rather, we think we do. In fact, linguists assure us, less than 10 percent of what we actually communicate comes from the words we use; the rest comes from our gestures and body language, and from our tone of voice and inflection. The assumption that we always communicate with words can be a detriment to the development of body language, the senses, and intuition. We can also sing or dance, sculpt, draw, or paint our prayers.

When We Use Words

However, the majority of persons do tend to use words first when they come to prayer. Words, voiced or unvoiced, help us to make confession, to offer praise and thanksgiving, and to name needs. While profoundly deep and effective prayers are possible without a spoken word, some people may not be sure they have truly prayed rightly for themselves or others unless they use words. Certainly those being prayed for in a healing ministry are often helped by hearing the words.

Thoughts formed as words in the mind or spoken from the lips are powerful. Vocalized words go out on the breath according to the will, to set in motion the intention of the heart.

Here are some general reminders about use of words in prayer for ourselves or with others, whether spoken aloud or not.

1. Pray **positively.** Do not energize the negative condition or the diagnosis. (It may turn out to be wrong!)
2. Pray **affirmatively.** Recall what God is willing and able to do.
3. Pray **simply.** Elaborate and long speech can weaken prayer. Jesus' prayers for healing were pithy!
4. Pray **naturally.** Use language that is you.
5. Pray **lovingly.** Without love, prayer is but the sounding of a "noisy gong or a clanging cymbal" (1 Corinthians 13:1).
6. Pray **confidently.** Prayer without faith lacks power.

In spoken prayer for another who is present, choose language, images, or style that will make the prayer comfortable and helpful to that person. When using names that refer to God (Father, Mother, Divine Parent, Ever-Loving One...) or images (Light, Rock, Hen, Eagle, Shepherd...), try to ensure that no barrier is set up which may interfere with the harmony of the connection between the two of you.

In preparing his disciples for the persecution they would face in their ministry, Jesus assured them:

> *...do not worry about how you are to speak*
> *or what you are to say;*
> *for what you are to say will be given to you at that time;*
> *for it is not you who speak,*
> *but the Spirit of your Father speaking through you.*
> (Matthew 10:19-20)

When we allow the Spirit to take control, what is helpful to speak will be given to us.

When We Use Imagery

The kinds of images we work with have a profound influence on us.

A handsome prince had a crooked back. He was sad, for his condition kept him from doing what he longed to do. His father, the king, commissioned the best sculptor in the land to make a statue of the prince, portraying him not with a crooked back but a straight one. The statue was placed in the prince's private garden. Each day, as he sat in the garden, the prince gazed upon the statue. As he did, his heart beat faster, and he imagined seeing himself tall and straight like the statue.

As the months passed, the people began to notice that the prince's back did not seem as crooked as it had been. When the prince heard that, his heart beat even faster.

Now he began to spend hours studying the statue and meditating upon it. Then one day he became aware that he himself was standing as tall and straight as the statue!

Imaging is a helpful form of prayer for many people. It is powerful and effective, whether praying for oneself or for others.

Images may arise spontaneously, as word of knowledge, guidance, or as God's response. A colleague of healing, Gloria, writes,

> *In September of 1996, I started giving Therapeutic Touch treatments to a friend who had cancer return for the third time. My friend has had many significant imaging experiences during the treatments. Sometimes she has seen a white dove; but the most profound are the ones where she meets Jesus. The first time, Jesus came to her as she saw herself sitting on a rock beside the Sea of Galilee. He asked her to go for a walk with him. She told him she was in pain, and he said, "I know. That is why I am here to help you." On another occasion, she was having difficulty breathing, and was coughing frequently. But, during the treatment, her breathing became normal, and there was no coughing at all. It is now a year since the treatments began, and during the last few sessions, my friend has seen Jesus in the room with us. Doctors are now reporting that the cancer has not spread to her bones as they had expected, nor is she experiencing the level of pain or the nausea anticipated.*

The terms "visualization" and "imagery" are often used interchangeably. Some teachers of imagery tell their people what to think of – such as little "Pac-Man" microbes running around gobbling up cancer cells. I believe that we can find within ourselves the images we need for healing to occur. Visualization is consciously practicing the healing images we have discovered or created, allowing them to become more dominant in the mind.

Imagery works to facilitate healing in spirit, mind, or body, and to connect these aspects of the self. It provides a way for more of what is unconscious to become conscious. Images show us both our inner landscape and ways to change this landscape. Through imagery we can facilitate healing by replacing old, painful images with more nurturing and empowering ones.

Much body work practiced by therapists uses imagery. For example, a client may identify and locate a certain emotion in the body, and allow an image of it to emerge. Then, to facilitate the releasing and healing, energy work is done in that area of the body or with that image. This can be a means of prayer in which one engages alone under the protection and guidance of the Holy Spirit, but is usually most effective with the assistance of a trained other.

Some doctors use imagery for pain and stress management, for treating cancer and other diseases, for aiding the human body in its healing processes. Imagery alters the biochemistry of the brain.

Imagery can be literal, like the prince gazing upon the statue until he grew into its likeness, but it is more often symbolic. Every culture and religion has symbols. The Christian religion has its own set of images with symbolic meaning: cross, crucifix, light, water, baptismal shell, font, lamb, bread, wine, open Bible, votive candle, statue, tree of life, to name just a few. Light and water imagery is not confined to the Christian religion; however, these seem to be symbols which we share universally. To hold any of these as images in the mind is to be in touch with the power and the healing that can be released through them.

These images may find expression through a variety of media. An image may emerge under our hands as we hold a piece of clay while meditating upon the passage. Or an image may be sculpted through a position taken by the body. In symbol, drawing, clay, or body, the images may emerge in an evolving procession.

Icons can also be used profitably for Christian meditation. Icons are special images, visual expressions painted under the inspiration of the Holy Spirit. As such they have power, as does the written word. Henri Nouwen's *Behold the Beauty of the Lord: Praying with Icons* describes icons as a means of accessing "through the gate of the visible, the mystery of the invisible." He says that icons can lead us into the inner room of prayer, and bring us "close to the heart of God."

Protestants often feel a fear, instilled by the Reformation, that this is an unfaithful practice. But we are slowly overcoming this inhibition. We have come beyond what separated us, and are beginning again to appreciate the use of icons for focusing in prayer, as the Orthodox and Roman Catholic Churches have long done.

An "archetype" is a symbol of the collective unconscious. C. G. Jung, the Swiss psychiatrist, said, "There is an archetypal reality that has a life of its own." Archetypal symbols undergird the structure of the psyche – symbols such as the baby, old woman, hero, savior, bear, serpent, or eagle. These may make themselves known at certain times in our psychological development through night dreams or "waking dreams," times of receptive imaging prayer. The Christ archetype may surface in these times as well.

We can use imagery in praying the scripture, too. In this approach we do not come to a passage analytically to study its meaning and context, but in a prayerful, open and receptive mode, using intuition more than intellect. In this type of meditation, we set our minds free, under the protection and guidance of the Holy Spirit. We invite and allow fresh meaning to arise from within, as senses and imagination combine.

The content and symbols of the passage itself provide a structure for this process. How often we have said when meditating upon a very familiar passage of scripture, "I've never seen or thought or been moved by this before!" If you have not prayed the scripture before, you will find a guide in Appendix C.

Directing Our Thoughts

There is, as well, an active kind of Christian prayer in which we take responsibility for our thinking and imaging. Paul wrote to the Philippians,

> *Whatever is true, whatever is honorable, whatever is just,*
> *whatever is pure, whatever is pleasing, whatever is*
> *commendable, if there is any excellence and if there is anything*
> *worthy of praise, think about these things.*
> (Philippians 4:8)

In these words, he teaches us that it matters what we think, particularly what we hold in our minds.

Thoughts have energy. They are energy; they are little bits of information going out to land somewhere, and create. Even as the universe was a great thought in the mind of God before it came to be, so form follows our thought.

Each of us is an image held in the mind of God; God sees us as we can become and loves us as we are. God expects us to see ourselves according to that image too. When our minds are turned to the potential that is God's image for us, we are tuned to the blueprint level, to the spiritual template for our lives. In resonance with this image of ourselves, we put ourselves in touch with the power that actualizes this potential in the physical. When we *"set our mind on things that are above"* as Paul tells the Colossians to do (3:2a), we resonate with the power that brings into being things of highest good and beauty, things of eternal worth.

Images or mental pictures that we hold in our minds have an energy of their own. This energy is itself a form of prayer. What we visualize will materialize!

If we see ourselves as healthy, we will promote health. If we see ourselves as skillful and capable in a certain area, we will become so. If we see ourselves as lovable and loving, we will find ourselves given opportunities to experience love. If we see ourselves as a beloved child of God, we will be empowered to love as one.

In order to bring into being that which is not yet, we must image it as if it already were. Jesus taught that if we pray with faith and in love, believing we have received what we asked for (imaged), it will be ours.

Praying by Listening

Many persons speak of prayer as communication, but spend all their prayer time talking. To communicate we must listen as well as speak. We receive God's responses as we go about our daily affairs; as I have said, prayer is being attentive to God all the time. Yet there is a place in prayer life for intentional listening. We can too often miss that still small voice within, in the activity, busyness and noise of our everyday world. To hear, we must quiet not only our speaking but the myriad thoughts and voices that chase through our minds. We need to come to the quiet center of our souls, and be attentive.

To pray effectively for others, we need to be able to listen to them. We practice those skills by learning to listen – to our own thoughts, to our bodies, and to the movement of God's spirit in us.

Praying for Others

Tennyson wrote a moving call to intercessory prayer, that is, prayer for others, in *The Passing of Arthur:*

> *If thou shouldst never see my face again,*
> *Pray for my soul.*
> *More things are wrought by prayer*
> *Than this world dreams of.*

Wherefore, let thy voice
Rise like a fountain for me night and day.
For what are men better than sheep or goats
That nourish a blind life within the brain,
If, knowing God, they lift not hands of prayer
Both for themselves and those who call them friend?
For so the whole round earth is every way
Bound by gold chains about the feet of God.

In intercessory prayer, we follow the example of Jesus. In those long nights he spent alone in prayer, his prayers were surely not only for himself but for his disciples, his friends and family, the lost and sick among whom he taught and ministered, and the world his Father loved. Jesus' teaching concerning intercessory prayer begins with the words, *"Our Father..."* Not *my* father, but *our* father – parent for us all. It continues throughout as a communal prayer of praise and petition.

Jesus' whole being breathed his prayers for the sick in spirit, mind or body. When his disciples were frightened in a storm, he bade the winds be still. In John 17, he prayed that we, like his disciples, might be protected and equipped for intercession in the world, by our oneness with him. Jesus himself became a prayer of intercession upon the cross – the most complete prayer that could be offered.

Paul's ministry, like Jesus', was of intercession. In writing to the Romans Paul said,

For God, whom I serve with my spirit by announcing the gospel
of his Son, is my witness that without ceasing
I remember you always in my prayers. (Romans 1:9)

And he instructed the church in its ministry of prayer:

I urge that supplications, prayers, intercessions,
and thanksgivings be made for everyone.
(1 Timothy 2:1)

And James' instructions could not be clearer:

...pray for one another that you may be healed... (James 5:16)

We are placed in community as members of families, churches, and society, that we may care for one another, and together be a corporate expression of God's love. This includes holding before God in prayer the needs of individuals, groups of persons, whole communities, and the world, as Jesus did.

A First Resort

You have probably heard people say, "There's nothing more we (or the doctors) can do. We'll just have to pray." You may have said it yourself! Often this sounds as if prayer must be a last resort, instead of a first action we take.

Such a statement implicitly supports the idea that human knowledge and skill can solve and cure anything. It speaks of human pride and the sin of self-sufficiency. God has a way of reminding us that as children, even mature daughters and sons, we are not independent. Preacher William Temple said,

> When I pray for my friends, coincidences happen to them. When I cease to pray, the coincidences cease.

Although this may sound arrogant, it is not. It's an observation, a delight in the effects of prayer. Prayer charges the environment with spiritual energy, creating new channels through which the power of God can flow.

Perhaps the reason we tend to pray last instead of first is because of our doubts and questions. Those who pray for another will not necessarily have all their wonderings put to rest. But they must have a measure of faith, albeit the size of a grain of mustard seed. Jesus tells us what even that much faith can do! Intercessory prayers can be in word or silence, image, sigh or touch. But in whatever way we ask for another, we ask with the confidence of faith.

Richard Foster, author of *Coming Home: A Prayer Journal,* says that if we truly love people, we will desire for them far more than we can give them. And this will lead us to prayer, for intercession is a way of loving others.

Today in many churches there is a renewed interest in prayer groups and prayer chains. More and more persons are answering the call to love others in this way. Sometimes people may feel they have been given what is called a "prayer burden" by God, meaning that they sense that God wants to do a special work through their prayers on behalf of another. It takes what Paul called "devotion to our prayers" to continue faithfully in prayer until there is a sense of having "prayed through," but there does come a moment when it feels that the prayer burden has been lifted.

All of us are called to the ministry of intercession, but for some it is their particular calling. As we do the holy work of intercession, we hold in our heart the assurance of Paul to the Corinthians:

> *Since it is by God's mercy that we are engaged in this ministry,*
> *we do not lose heart.* (2 Corinthians 4:1)

It is God's work, God's mercy and grace, and God's power that accomplish great things. Our responsibility is to pray, and to leave the outcome to God.

What Does "In Jesus' Name" Mean?

The expression *"to believe in the name of Jesus"* is found only in the writings of John, where it occurs five times. The phrases *"to believe in the name of Jesus"* and *"to believe in Jesus"* clearly mean the same thing. "Name" in the Bible signifies essential being. We are to offer our prayers with the same mind and heart that was, and is, in Jesus. We are to pray in the Christ Spirit.

In speaking to people in the temple, Peter testified,

> *By faith in his [Jesus'] name, his name itself has made this man*
> *strong, whom you see and know; and the faith that is through*
> *Jesus has given him this perfect health in the presence of all of you.*
> (Acts 3:16)

In healing prayer, then, to pray "in Jesus' name" is to declare the authority of Jesus over the healing. To speak or act in someone's name is to act as the representative of that person, to participate in that person's authority. In her healing work, Rochelle has often noticed the clearing of blocks instantly, upon the use of the name of Jesus.

To pray with the confidence of Jesus that our prayers are heard, Christ must be in us. Writing to the Galatians, Paul says, *"...until Christ is formed in you"* (Galatians 4:19b). He also said,

> *Do you not know that your body is a temple of the Holy Spirit*
> *within you, which you have from God?* (1 Corinthians 6:19)

We are drawn to ask, is Christ "being formed in me?" In other words, is the Spirit of Jesus being given the freedom to pray through me?

We pray that the Spirit, nature, mind and heart of Christ grow strong in us. By our personal, ongoing relationship with Jesus Christ in the depths of our own soul we are prepared for effective intercession, prepared to ask boldly, and to say to God, as Jesus did, "I know you always hear my prayers." The apostle John assures us.

> *This is the boldness we have in him, that if we ask anything*
> *according to his will, he hears us.* (1 John 5:14)

Yet we know that in our humanity, there is in most of us still a struggle of the ego for control, still some personal block which affects our prayer. We are still in the making. And so, not being perfectly united with the mind and heart of Christ, we cannot presume to know the will of God for another's life. Fortunately, God provided for us in our weakness, by giving us the Holy Spirit who intercedes through us.

> *The Spirit helps us in our weakness; for we do not know how to*
> *pray as we ought, but that very Spirit intercedes with sighs too*
> *deep for words. And God, who searches the heart, knows what is*
> *the mind of the Spirit, because the Spirit intercedes for the saints*
> *according to the will of God.* (Romans 8:26-27)

Persistence Pays

Whatever the mode of prayer, persistence may be necessary. Healing is very often a process. Even Jesus prayed more than once in healing a blind man at Bethsaida.

> *...when he had put saliva on his eyes and laid his hands on him,*
> *he asked him, "Can you see anything?" And the man looked up*
> *and said, "I can see people but they look like trees, walking." Then*
> *Jesus laid his hands on his eyes again...and his sight was restored.*
> (Mark 8:23b-25)

Jesus himself taught that persistence makes a difference. For example, after telling the story of one who goes to a friend at midnight asking for loaves of bread, Jesus says,

I tell you, even though he will not get up and give him anything
because he is his friend, at least because of his persistence he will
get up and give him whatever he needs. (Luke 11:8)

Persistence proves faith, and faith enables persistence. God knows the way and the time for the highest good to break through. We soften the clay of condition and situation with our prayer until it is malleable, ready to be reshaped "in the fullness of time" by the Master Potter's loving hands.

But does God need our prayers? Isn't God capable of everything?

The answer to both questions, we believe, is "yes." God is omnipotent. But God has also chosen to limit God's self so that we might learn to cooperate with the laws of the universe, the laws that sustain our lives and our planet. Because of those self-imposed limits, God expects and counts on our prayers for others and for creation and wants us to be partners in bringing about the fullness of the reign of Christ upon earth. Each of us may say, "Who, me?" And God answers, "Why not you?" As we embody the light and love of Christ, we emit harmonious vibrations into the environment of our families, communities, and the earth. Such spiritual energy is healing and lifegiving.

We make this contribution first by who we "be," and secondarily by what we "do." In this sense, we *become* prayer.

Prayer for Guidance

Sometimes fog envelops a ship's deck at water level, and yet leaves the top mast clear. Then a sailor goes aloft, to see what the helmsman on deck cannot see. So prayer sends the soul aloft, lifts it above the doubt and disbelief that befog us, and gives us a chance to see which way to steer.

We need to go aloft, so to speak, because being skilled in technique carries us only so far. We can say the words, but unless we train ourselves to also be sensitive to the Spirit, we can miss guidance when it is given.

This training we can do in our everyday life. When we rise each morning and offer the day to God, we encourage the Spirit to move with us through the day, guiding us along. Not only in big things, like making important decisions, but in little ways, nudging us to go here, stop there, make this call, read that.

Cultivating a life of prayer, meditation, and contemplation is not selfish. It prepares us to do our ministry in the world in the name of Jesus. Thomas Merton says, "Contemplation gives insights beyond analysis."

Then, when we come to pray for or minister to another, we find we are guided. Words come to our lips; our hands move almost without our volition. Such experiences are amazing but not surprising when we give ourselves to God, heart and mind, word and hand, to be vehicles of grace and blessing.

When we let go of concerns about how we will perform and what we will say, and lift our attention to the One who called us to ministry and who equips us by the Spirit, we will find ourselves guided in wondrous ways. We may hear ourselves praying about things we have not been told and could not have known ourselves. Or we may receive an intuitive knowing of how to proceed with the ministry.

Following this guidance becomes easier as we learn to trust the knowing as a gift of the Spirit.

Prayers of Protection

If you intend to offer the ministry of healing prayer to others, you need to prepare by praying protection for yourself, for the others working with you, and for the ministry about to begin. When we press into the spiritual realm with our prayer, we can expect resistance. There will be a push back in some form. But a muscle, for example, becomes stronger when it has a resistance against which to work. Jesus experienced the full force of this resistance in the wilderness, and it served to prepare him for what lay ahead in his ministry.

However we wish to name the dark powers of the universe, Christian prayer activates an opposing energy. Therefore, we *"put on the whole armor of God"* (Ephesians 6:10-17). With the protection of the Holy Spirit and God's angels and the exercise of our faith, we are able to be strong, confident, and safe as we do our ministry. As we lift up the name of Jesus, and pray in the Spirit, we resonate with the highest spiritual energy and vibration of the universe. To pray for the protection of the Christ is to place around ourselves this special energy through which nothing of lower energy can penetrate. We can image this protection as light, or a ring of fire, or a warm blanket wrapped around us by Jesus.

In preparing oneself, one can offer a simple prayer or use words like this affirmation of faith.

The Light of God surrounds and protects me,
the Love of God enfolds and fills me,
the Spirit of God inspires and guides me with all Truth.

Then, trusting in God's faithfulness, one can begin to minister to the other from a centered, protected place.

At the close of the prayer for healing, whether by word and/or touch, it is wise to pray for the protection of the Holy Spirit around the recipient again. This can be easily included at the time of giving thanks to God who heals. It is like a seal upon the work that God has done in the time of prayer ministry.

Often the other person does not know how or why to do this. Wisdom is needed, to discern whether or not to talk about the need for this protection, and whether to pray aloud or silently. But this important step in completing the ministry is often unwisely neglected, forgotten, or discounted. In public church services or prayers for healing, liturgical acts accomplish this closure – for example, in the Benediction.

Hindrances to Prayer

There can be hindrances to prayer in the outer environment, or in the soul. Even Jesus had this experience in his hometown.

> *He could do no deed of power there,*
> *except that he laid his hands on a few sick people and cured them.*
> *And he was amazed at their unbelief.* (Mark 6:5-6a)

In Nazareth, the hindrance was the prevailing mood of unbelief, the attitude of the hometown folks toward Jesus. We can experience similar hindrances as we pray within a work or social scene, within a family, or a church. Negativity can interfere with prayer and healing.

Of lesser import, but also having an effect, are interruptions and excessive noise. It is often difficult, inadvisable, and sometimes even impossible, to continue vocal prayer in such circumstances. It would probably be best to pray silently.

In prayer, the hindrances can also be "us"! Jesus often posed a penetrating question to those who came to him. He asked the blind man, *"What do you want me to do for you?"* (Mark 10:51) To the man who had been lying for 38 years beside the pool waiting for healing, he said, *"Do you want to get well?"* (John 5:6) He might have taken their desires for granted. He may have known exactly what they needed. But *they* needed to know and voice that for themselves.

We too need to recognize that some persons, in their inmost being, may not really want to be well. Many people fear the unknown; they fear change, even good change. Having become used to a certain condition, they may have an unconscious resistance to becoming different. Such persons have an "investment" in their illness.

Illness can be used to manipulate one's environment, and the people in it. If the back problem went away, it might mean having to go back to work for the difficult boss. If the legs were better, it might mean the family would not "fetch and carry." If one were not bedridden, the family would not visit as often, and life would be more lonely.

Viewing illness as punishment is also a hindrance to becoming well. Unless this understanding of illness as punishment is removed, even if treatment brings about change, it will probably be temporary. The condition will in all likelihood return to its former state. In cases like these, Jesus spoke first to the person's inner condition, to remove the block.

Some persons may resist prayer because of an unwillingness to risk hoping. There is fear of unanswered prayer. Not to ask seems safer.

Praying obsessively may also be a hindrance. We need to "believe it, and leave it." Agnes Sanford, a pioneer of healing prayer ministry, taught that it is best to pray and then go about our other business. We may return again and again, but on each occasion, we must pray and then take our hands off, so to speak. In this way, we permit God's good to manifest itself as is best at that particular time.

The main hindrance, though, is almost always an unwillingness to surrender, to hand oneself and one's life over to God. Only when we do can God help us deal with the other hindrances that we know, and those that we may not know. By our asking, our choosing, our willingness, God is freed to do for us what God desires.

Seemingly Unanswered Prayer

Doubts and questions abound. Many Christians hesitate to pray for healing for themselves or others because they cannot be certain that God answers prayer. As a result, much of the work of prayer is often left undone, and the most powerful means of healing are often left untapped.

In the Sermon on the Mount, when Jesus clearly instructs his followers to "ask...seek...and knock," he promises a receiving, a finding, and an opening of a door.

Is there anyone among you who, if your child asks for bread,
will give a stone? Or if the child asks for fish, will give a snake?
If you then...know how to give good gifts to your children,
how much more will your Divine Parent give good things
to those who ask! (Matthew 7:9-11)

What then do we believe if God does not give us the bread or fish we ask for, but rather something else? Something that may even appear to us to be a stone or a snake?

Jesus assured us that God *always* makes a good and loving response. But if that response does not look like what we have decided it ought to, we may fail to see God has answered our prayer. When we predetermine the answer, we limit our ability to see the answer that does come. And often God's answers come in the most surprising ways!

A few years ago, my teenage son was looking for a summer job, with no success. For weeks I had been praying, fearful that in idleness he might "fall in with the wrong crowd." I did not want him to become like a boy down the street, who was more absent from school than present, who wore black leather with studs and an earring in his nose, and who had just lost his driving license. Then one evening, my son was in the driveway. The other boy came walking past the house. Having his ear tuned to the news on the street among the teens, the studs-and-leather boy had just heard of a job opening. He suggested my son get on it right away. My son applied, and got the job. His summer hours were filled; his mother's prayer had been answered through the most unlikely person! I had to do some praying for forgiveness of prejudices!

There are no unanswered prayers. God is absolutely faithful to supply all our deepest needs, but not necessarily our wants! P. T. Forsyth asserts, "God's great refusals were sometimes the true answers to our truest prayer."

God's answer to our prayer may be any of these:
- No, because I love you too much!
- No, not yet!
- Yes, I've been waiting for you to ask!
- Yes, but not as you expect!
- Yes, and more than you expect!

The biblical Letter to the Ephesians includes this prayer:

Now to God who by the power at work within us is able to
accomplish abundantly far more than all we can ask or
imagine...be glory in the church and in Christ Jesus...
(Ephesians 3:20-21)

On our part, we must pay attention to what we are really energizing in our prayer: faith or unbelief, need or want, what we perceive to be good or God's highest good. And we must be willing not only to trust God's ways, but to await God's timing.

We tend to expect God's answers to be overt and active, to bring a solution where there is a problem, or curing where there is illness. We attempt to say to God, as we say to each other: "Don't just stand there. Do something!"

Lynne, a clergy person, told of a pastoring experience:

I was to prepare a sermon on Exodus 17 – Moses striking the rock
to get water. I got out the commentary and read "Moses getting
water from the rock shows us how there is always a bend at the
end of the road." My anger flared. I had recently listened to the
story of one of "my" families where the mother of three children
had died of a kidney disease. Prayers were sent in abundance. For
the bereaved, to suggest there will be a bend at the end of the road
is to minimize their pain. It minimizes, too,
the evil of the crucifixion.

As I prepared my message, I wrestled with the experience of not
having prayers answered. I muttered to God about how unfair it is
that some are answered and some are not.

After Sunday worship – I had three services to do – I found myself
still angry with God. As I vigorously chopped vegetables for the
lunch salad, I said to God, "It really is a lousy system you know –
that some prayers are answered and some not." Deep within some
quiet center of my being came the words: "Why do I always have
to do something? Can't I just be there?"

My heart melted. My feelings of anger dissipated. How many
times had I said to a loved one, with my own heart grieving, "I
know I can't do anything, but I can be here for you." God was
offering me that same loving gift. I was honored.

We do not live in isolation but in community, connected and intertwined not only with each other but with all creation. While God's caring is individual and particular, it is also general and all-encompassing. Therefore, God's answers must reflect the divine wisdom and understanding of what is the ultimate highest good for all.

Indeed, God pours blessings upon us all the time, not just when we pray. Most of the time, God's goodness is more likely to go unnoticed. Not only in discerning God's answers to prayer, but at all times, our responsibility is to be open, sensitive, and responsive to God's presence and activity.

Healing of Inner Attitudes

Jesus captured an essential truth when he said,

> *You shall love the Lord your God with all your heart,*
> *and with all your soul, and with all your mind.*
> (Matthew 22:37)

If we have a negative concept of ourselves as healers, if we are pessimistic rather than hope-filled and expectant of good, and if we are critical or judgmental rather than lovingly accepting, these attitudes will affect more than our own well-being and energy. Consciously or unconsciously, they will affect others. Therefore we have a responsibility to examine ourselves. We pray as did the psalmist:

> *Search me, O God, and know my heart;*
> *test me and know my thoughts.*
> (Psalm 139:23)

In laying bare our own heart, mind, and motives before God, we ourselves will be increasingly transformed. We not only gain self-understanding, but understanding and compassion for others. And our inner attitudes will affect our prayer for and with others.

Jesus continued his summary of the Law with a second command: *"Love your neighbor as yourself."* To love oneself with a holy and healthy love means neither thinking more highly of ourselves than we ought and falling into pride, nor "putting ourselves down" and negating the unique gift of God that each one of us is.

Yet people are often willing to pray for others, but will hesitate to pray for themselves. They may think it is selfish to pray for themselves. They may not believe they are worthy to ask for their own needs. Without a healthy sense of self, a negative voice within may foster self-doubt and self-criticism. In one sense, none of us are "worthy" – we are all, to some extent, flawed and sinful people. But in God's eyes we are worthy; through Jesus, God has declared us accepted and forgiven.

Some are able to accept that assurance readily. For others, it is a lifetime journey. I remember being told countless times as a child, "Be good now!" The instruction implied that being good was something other than what I already was! It took years to come to accept that the words of Isaiah 43:4 were for me as for Israel:

You are precious in my sight…and I love you.

Pessimism

An unhealed self-concept can result in a pessimistic attitude toward one's own life, and toward life in the world in general.

If I do not believe I am worth much, my thoughts, speech and demeanor may resemble those of Eeyore, in *Winnie the Pooh*. On a sunny day, I will expect rain. If it doesn't rain today, I will expect it to rain tomorrow. My head and eyes will be as downcast as my thoughts. In fact, my whole body will sag. I will bring the rain into my own life and the life of others by my obvious attitude, my bearing, and my words. And, if I am Eeyore the Pessimist, I will not allow myself to be cheered either!

But if I am Pooh, I will expect wonderful adventures. I will expect to find honey, and to have friends! I may make many mistakes. But I will know life is about learning and loving and forgiving. I will look for "the good" in life, and I will find it! It may rain, but I will know the sun will come out again. So I will hum my little tune as I look for my next adventure, even if my hum is off-key.

If we know our worth as children of God, we have an inherited right to expect that all things will work together for good, not ill. The rain in life is intended to soften the ground of the soul, so that "the good" may take root and grow in us. We believe that the Spirit within enables us to control any pessimistic thoughts that may plague us from time to time, to bind and cast them out, and in their stead to affirm that "we have the mind of Christ."

Criticism

We tend to project onto others the criticisms we unconsciously direct toward ourselves, or the conditions that are unresolved, unforgiven, or unhealed within ourselves. If criticism has given us a negative self-image, we are vulnerable to projecting this pain outward.

We may think that our critical attitudes will remain undiscovered because they are hidden in our minds. But we are mistaken. Those attitudes can be encountered in the fields of energy; they will show in body language, in the tightness of muscles of face and torso, and in tone of voice.

To criticize is to make a judgment concerning another. An old Native proverb goes something like this: "Whoever would judge another, should first walk a mile in his moccasins." We have a similar adage cautioning about making hasty judgment: "Put yourself in their shoes!" I recall a woman in the throes of a marriage separation. She was experiencing much pain – not only because of the loss of her marriage dreams, her home, and separation from some of her children, but because of criticism from neighbors, friends, and church associates. They judged her to be either selfish or sinful, because she had initiated the family dissolution. With a mixture of sorrow and defensiveness, she said, "Let them first put their feet under my table, and their shoes under my bed, before they have anything to say!"

The Bible offers frequent cautions against hasty judgment. Jesus said,

> *Do not judge, so that you may not be judged!* (Matthew 7:1)
> *Do not judge by appearances...* (John 7:24a)
> *Let anyone among you who is without sin*
> *be the first to throw a stone.* (John 8:7b)

And Paul confirmed these cautions when he wrote to the church at Corinth,

> *Do not pronounce judgment before the time, before the Lord*
> *comes, who will bring to light the things now hidden in darkness*
> *and will disclose the purposes of the heart.* (1 Corinthians 4:5a)

Depression

Depression may well be the most common malaise of the inner life. It affects every facet of a person's being. Depression can range from a mild, passing condition born of fatigue, temporary illness, overwork, worry or other emotional state, to severe and chronic depression.

Like any other dis-ease of spirit, mind, and emotion, depression may have a physical cause. Depression may also result from loss, lack of love, fear, insecurity, or a sense of meaninglessness. In these instances, prayer for healing can release the love of Jesus into the life of suffering persons with profound beneficial effect. Body work is effective in releasing congestions of energy and re-establishing its flow. Spiritual and/or psychological counseling may be required. If the depression has its source in spiritual oppression, then prayer for deliverance in the name of Jesus can scatter this power.

Many today suffer from what is called "clinical depression." When the chemistry of the body is out of balance, for whatever reason, depression results. Both doctors and patients struggle valiantly today to alter the chemistry through drugs, to discover what works for a person, and what will enable the patient to function in life.

Love and caring, emotional and spiritual support, are crucial gifts the church can offer. Prayers of acceptance and assurance encourage persons with this clinical disorder. Healing touch, from hugs to treatments, can be given with helpful results. But if we believe anything about prayer, we must believe that God can affect the chemistry of a brain. And so we pray for healing with all the faith and love in us. To pray, we do not need to know what upset the chemistry in the first place. We pray expectantly, positively, and persistently, realizing that only God knows all the factors of the person's genetic and spiritual blood streams. We simply pray believing in God's healing will and power, and rest our prayers there.

Emotions and Memories

Not all the problems for which we seek healing are current. The past can continue to influence us.

Deepak Chopra is a medical doctor, a scientist, and the author of numerous best-selling books. In *Ageless Body, Timeless Mind,* he says that in less than one year, 90 percent of the atoms in the body are replaced, the skeleton changes every three months, and the lining of the stomach every five days. He asks us to consider why, then, 90 percent of the thoughts we have today we had yesterday. He suggests it is because we are "stuck in our thinking."

In one startling statement, Chopra says, "The tormentor today is myself left over from yesterday." Like fellow author Wayne Dyer, he argues that we must learn to use our memories, not allow memories to use us. We must untie the strings that have been tying up our awareness. Dyer, in his book *The Sacred*

Self, uses the metaphor of life as a boat; he says that we live under the delusion that the wake is driving the boat! We allow what happened yesterday to drive our life today.

Experiences and memories of the past can and often do bind our thinking and feeling responses. David Hilton, M.D. and a former staff member of the Christian Medical Commission of the World Council of Churches, warns of the effect of emotional, mental, spiritual, or relational distress on the physical being:

> *The most important dimension to health is the spiritual. Even in the midst of poverty, some people stay well, while among the world's affluent many are chronically ill. Why? Medical science is beginning to affirm that one's beliefs and feelings are the ultimate tools and powers for healing. Unresolved guilt, anger, resentment, and meaninglessness are found to be the greatest suppressors of the body's powerful, health-controlling immune system, while loving relationships in community are among its strongest augmenters. Those in harmony with the Creator, the earth, and their neighbors not only survive tragedy and suffering best, but grow stronger in the process.*

We get "sick at heart" from grief, "hard-hearted" from anger, or "cold-hearted" from fear. But our emotions may evoke even more serious responses. We can die of a broken heart, and shattered dreams. We can die from loneliness, and from meaninglessness in life.

Emotions have been called "psychic motors." The word "emotion" comes from the Latin *movere,* to move. Emotions move us. In anger, the face often flushes and muscles become tense. In fear, the palms sweat, the stomach knots, the mouth becomes dry, the body trembles. Even recalling those emotions from the past can result in the same reaction. People relive the trauma of a car accident, a break-in, a slight or insult, over and over again.

It is not the passing thought, the flash of anger or other emotion, that does us harm. In fact these can be a healthy release. But the recurring emotions that we entertain and harbor, that we dwell upon, that we refuse to release, can and will harm us. When we turn negative thoughts around and around in the mind, when we rehearse hurts and grievances, the effect can register chronically as physical disease.

There are biblical precedents for this insight. The psalmist connects his grief and emotional anguish to his well-being:

My life is spent with sorrow, and my years with sighing; my
strength fails because of my misery, and my bones waste away.
(Psalm 31:10)

Proverbs – the folk-wisdom of the Hebrew people – often affirms that an intense emotion, a compulsion, causes a decaying of health in the body:

A tranquil mind gives life to the flesh,
but passion makes the bones rot. (Proverbs 14:30)
A cheerful heart is a good medicine,
but a downcast spirit dries up the bones. (Proverbs 17:22)
Hope deferred makes the heart sick... (Proverbs 13:12a)

Ecclesiastes 7:9 describes the long-lasting effects of emotions:

Do not be quick to anger, for anger lodges in the bosom of fools.

All of these affirm that health of mind, heart and spirit are essential to the health of the body. Psychological and spiritual counseling release the blocks to the body's own restorative power. The use of touch, as in Healing Touch, Therapeutic Touch, or Reiki, can be part of this releasing process to clear congestions in the energy field or to fill weak places. Prayer is a powerful agency for this work.

Hurts of the past lodged in our hearts, minds, and bodies often need spiritual work to bring healing. One way to the "healing of the memories" – a phrase used by Agnes Sanford – involves asking Jesus to walk back with us into the wounded places of our lives, places where we experienced abuse, rejection, or abandonment, places which have bound us in the darkness and distress of painful memories. As we open ourselves in prayer, Jesus can and does go back with us to bring healing, for Jesus is not bound by space and time as we are.

We do not always choose the time for such a journey ourselves. One time, I was on a silent retreat. Awakening early one morning, resting and meditating in my bed, an image of a fetus in a womb suddenly came to mind. At the same time, my body was drawn into a fetal position. I knew the little unborn one was me in my mother's womb.

My mother, long deceased, was a loving, caring parent. But she was private, reserved in verbal and physical affection, a product of her own era and strict, religious upbringing. After having two boys, five years apart, there was a space of nine years, and then she was unexpectedly pregnant again.

Although we had never discussed such things, I realized in that moment that mother must have been upset and anxious, even frightened, by this late pregnancy. She was already in her 40s, working hard on the farm as the family struggled to keep bills paid in years of depression. Perhaps unconsciously, she had feelings of not wanting this child. These thoughts would not be acceptable to her, and perhaps even made her feel guilty. The fetus picked up these emotions in her womb, and resulted in a baby who was fretful and nervous, had digestive problems, and cried a lot. Or so I have been told!

It all came clear in that moment, lying in bed at the retreat. I got up, took my journal – long a private friend – and began to write, amid tears, a conversation with my mother. I felt an almost overpowering sense of love for my mother, and a sense of her spirit with me as I wrote. I wrote of my love for her, and of my understanding of her situation and feelings when she had been carrying me in her womb. The loving presence of the living Christ in the room was almost palpable.

Later, I shared this experience with the retreat director. We prayed together. Much emotional healing resulted from this experience. God's timing had been perfect.

When emotional or spiritual wounding has caused physical illness, the point of entry for healing may be through prayer and/or touch.

Lynda had been experiencing physical heart problems, and was filled with fears as she awaited test results. One day as Lynda and I were praying in my home, I felt moved to lay my hand gently on Lynda's upper chest, with Lynda's permission, as we prayed for inner healing of heart, mind and spirit. I felt as if her chest had gone concave during our prayer.

When I asked Lynda to write her experience, for this book, she wrote,

> *I could feel her gentle touch. But as the prayer proceeded, I began*
> *to feel a hand enter my body, going through my flesh and bones*
> *until it came to rest upon my heart. There it gently rested, and*
> *then left in the same manner. Not only had I been able to feel the*
> *hand enter and leave, I could envision it!*
> *Flora's gentle touch had not changed.*

I knew it had been the hand of God.
The test results were not perfect, but the peace that I had experi-
enced through that touch was enough to take the worry away. It
left me not only with a new sense of God's power and love, but
with a heart that was more gentle and loving.

Grief

Grief after loss is actually the beginning of healing. Not to experience the pain is to be shut off from oneself. And the unfolding stages of grief are also natural and necessary. To state briefly a subject on which many books have been written, grief has three main stages:

- **Denial,** a stage of shock and numbness, and vacillation between fantasy and reality. One feels, "It can't be true!"
- **Despair,** a stage of deep sadness, where anger or tears may be alternately ventilated, possibly with depression, very low energy, and a struggle with guilt or self-condemnation.
- **Acceptance,** a stage of knowing that in spite of loss, life must and does go on, and that there is still love to give and receive.

In his book, *Don't Take My Grief Away*, Doug Manning describes grief like a cut finger. It is numb before it bleeds, bleeds before it hurts, hurts until it begins to heal, then forms a scab and itches until finally, the scab is gone and a small scar is left where once there was a wound. He says that grief is the deepest wound a person can have. Like a cut finger, it goes through stages and leaves a scar.

From my son's death, I know that these stages do not follow in neat steps. They are constantly interwoven. I move back and forth, returning again and again to an early place in the process, just when I thought maybe I was moving on! The slightest reminder of the loss – even no reminder at all – can bring back denial or anger or debilitating pain. But gradually, very gradually, the pain dulls at each revisiting. And I do grow stronger, and better able to integrate the reality of my changed world.

But it is easy to get stuck somewhere along the journey to acceptance of this changed life. Sometimes I have needed help to move on. This help has come through the love and prayers of others in my life, and through the laying on of hands in healing services. It has come through receiving bioenergy treatments to break up congested areas, to restore the flow of energy through the whole being, and generally to assist in re-establishing the balance necessary for wellness.

Unresolved grief, like unconfessed guilt, unhealed hurt, unforgiven failures, chronic anger, and perpetual fear, weaken the immune system. They will surely make us sick physically, as well as mentally, emotionally, spiritually – and possibly relationally. Confusion, depression, anxiety and apathy can be signs. People may say – revealingly – that they feel "dispirited." The whole being moves into a state of lowered spiritual energy.

By turning our eyes toward Jesus, alive and with us, and trusting in his power to heal, we are moved toward healing. We surrender to God who ever reaches toward us with comforting, sustaining arms. Opening up one's inner being, and offering all the emotions – pain, anger, doubt, the whole works – to the One who knows the pain of loss, allows the Spirit to do the work we cannot do for ourselves.

Forgiveness

For the health of body, mind and spirit, we need to give and receive the grace of forgiveness. Sunday by Sunday we make our communal confession and hear an assurance of pardon. We recognize together our participation in the sin of the world, and we receive the word of the gospel. If the liturgy allows sufficient time in silence for private confession as well, we are blessed.

However, often we pray what is on the surface and gloss over the emotions in our depths. Or these emotions may be too intense to unearth in a few moments. The guilt, hurt, or abuse may have been pushed down too long, or buried too far in the unconscious. Then we find ourselves driven by unnamed powers.

But God knows them. And God wants what is in our inmost heart brought into the light, so that it can be healed. As the Psalms say,

> *You have set our iniquities before you,*
> *our secret sins in the light of your countenance.* (Psalm 90:8)
> *Create in me a clean heart, O God,*
> *and put a new and right spirit within me...*
> *Restore to me the joy of your salvation,*
> *and sustain in me a willing spirit.* (Psalm 51:10,12)

We too can make our confession and receive the forgiveness we long for, by writing or speaking to God in private. Receiving prayer ministry from another can also be very helpful.

We who do prayer ministry must be ready to hear the confession of another, to unblock the path to healing. We must be ready to speak the word of forgiveness in Christ's name, and to affirm God's love and grace. Sometimes work with a trained therapist or counselor is necessary to unearth and deal with root causes.

Jesus cared more about people's suffering, as a result of the sin in their lives, than about the sin itself. Though he knew that guilt was making people sick, he did not berate them for their sin. He simply offered forgiveness.

Forgiveness and assurance of pardon enable healing from the spiritual dimension. Without forgiveness, there is no peace; without peace, wellness cannot be maintained. We can choose to forgive or not, to receive the gift of God's forgiveness or not. If we refuse forgiveness, we become endangered at all levels of our own being. The writer of the biblical Letter to the Hebrews offered this advice:

> *Pursue peace with everyone...*
> *See to it that no one fails to obtain the grace of God;*
> *that no root of bitterness springs up and causes trouble...*
> (Hebrews 12:14-15)

Jesus' teachings are very clear on forgiveness. He knew that only love can heal us and free us.

> *Forgive and you will be forgiven.* (Luke 6:37c)
> *Love your enemies and pray for those who persecute you...*
> (Matthew 5:44)

Prayer at a Distance

At some point in our prayer journey, we have all prayed for someone at a distance and wondered if it made any difference. We have prayed for a situation in a distant place in the world and wondered if it did any good. Even when we hear of an improvement in a person's condition or in a situation, we still wondered if our prayer contributed to the change, or if it would have happened anyway.

Such questions have no answer, apart from the conviction of our faith. But scientific research and prayer experiments today are adding to our assurance, teaching us that, yes, we can pray with effectiveness at a distance. And, yes, our prayers make a difference. Wayne, who has made special study of the scientific evidence for healing, documented some of these instances in Chapter 7.

As with all intercessory prayer, prayer at a distance begins with loving concern. Through love we are connected both with God and the person for whom we pray.

Mental pictures are helpful. We can image ourselves in the presence of the receiver, becoming energetically joined through love. As we continue to fill our mind with faith, hope, expectancy and love, we image the recipient bathed in the healing white light of God which cleanses, clears, rejuvenates and balances the energies.

Or we can send healing energy to the other through word or image, remembering not to impose our will, but desiring God's highest good. We can think of the words of our prayer as pieces of information sent into the energy field of the other. Therefore the intention and expression in words must be positive and faith-filled. But it need not be definitive, unless we are very certain of the leading of the Spirit. If a limb is broken, of course we can image it healed. Or if a person is grieving, we can image Jesus with arms around him or her. But if a person is depressed, we should avoid imaging a specific cause that requires curing; we can leave that up to God.

Scientific experiments indicate that we can either
enhance or inhibit healing by our attitudes. Do we also,
in a ministry of healing, need to be aware of negative energies?
Flora Litt *explores the reality of demons and angels.*

9

The Shadow Side

In a recent issue of *Psychology Today*, Larry Dossey, M.D., asked the question, "Can Prayer Harm?" He asserted that prayer has a shadow side. Negative beliefs and expectations can cause harm.

As an example, he cited a British study, conducted with the patients' consent, in which patients with stomach cancer were given a placebo (a sugar pill) instead of a chemotherapy drug they thought they were taking. They developed the same reactions they would have had to chemotherapy! One-third developed nausea, one-fifth vomiting, and approximately one-third lost their hair.

Dossey also reported a direct correlation between the positive or negative expectations of researchers and the effectiveness of vitamin E on angina patients. Similarly, other research suggests it is possible for persons to affect the growth of bacteria and fungi at a distance of up to 15 miles by mental concentration. Can persons be similarly affected by the nature and quality of thought projected toward them?

In fact, we affect each other constantly. We have all, at one time or another, had the experience of our inner or physical condition changing in the company of another, perhaps just by connecting with them on the phone or in thought. In the presence of someone depressed, angry, or negative, we find ourselves becoming infected by their mental/emotional condition or attitude. Or we find our own bleak mood suddenly lifted by encountering someone else's buoyant spirit. This happens without any conscious thought being sent toward us!

I vividly recall an instance when a woman – yes, in the church – was furiously angry and vengeful toward me. After an initial verbal attack, the woman turned away at any sight of me. I felt the injustice in every part of my being. My best efforts at reconciliation were refused; this was heartbreaking. But I remembered that both Jesus and Paul advised prayer at such times:

> *Pray for whose who persecute you.* (Matthew 5:44)
> *Bless those who persecute you;*
> *bless and do not curse them.* (Romans 12:14)

It was not easy to pray for love and God's highest good for my attacker, but I did it. In doing so, I found relief for the knots in my stomach, my sleeplessness, and my troubled spirit.

Even so, during several weeks following, a heavy and agitating wave of darkness would roll over me, without any reference to what I was doing at the time. It was so strong that it drained me; it was debilitating. Gradually over months this lessened, but still I had to cling to Jesus' promise to be with me. Repeatedly, I had to pray forgiveness and love toward the one who I felt might be directing negativity toward me.

Was it all in my own mind? Or could it really have been the intentionally negative thought-vibrations coming toward me?

I do believe that intensely negative thought can be considered negative prayer. In our culture, we do not stick pins in dolls, practice negative voodoo arts, or put curses upon one another. But neither are we immune from offering, probably unconsciously, what could be considered negative prayer. We energize what we consider to be our right, success, promotion, or gain at the expense of another. We send out unloving, angry, jealous thoughts toward another.

In a conflict, both sides may pray to defeat their opponent. Both sides prayed to win the Gulf War, at the expense of countless lives on the other side. In Jerusalem, Muslims, Jews, and Christians all pray for their own peace at the expense of the peace of Jerusalem. In Ireland, Roman Catholics and Protestants pray against one another at the expense of peace for all.

I smile at the story told of a woman terrified by an extremely rough airplane flight. When the plane landed, she pushed past the flight attendant and charged into the airport, demanding a refund on the rest of her ticket. She would go no further, although she had not reached her destination.

The attendant asked why she was leaving the plane. The woman reported the terrible flight, saying, "I was praying constantly to get that plane on the ground!"

The pilot, who had followed her in, overheard her comment. Stepping up beside her, he said, "I wish you had not been doing that! I was praying constantly to keep that plane in the air!"

When our intention in prayer is to be an agent of God's healing work, and when we offer prayer from a loving heart with faith in God's highest good, then our prayer will surely have good effect. But when we pray for a specific outcome, we may be unwittingly working against God's highest good. A minister once asked me, gently, about my prayers for my children: "Flora, are you praying for *your* will to be done? Are you getting in the way of what *God* wants for your children?"

Any time we presume to know what is best in another's life, and pray for that, we may be praying at cross-purposes with God. Just as one vote may nullify another in an election, one prayer may block another. For example, if one partner in an extremely difficult marriage is asking God for a way to be released, while a well-meaning parent prays that the marriage continue no matter what, an impasse restricts relief and resolution.

Evil Spirits

In inviting the participation of other spiritual energies in our lives, we must be careful. Just as we would not invite any unknown person to share the intimacy of our human life, neither do we invite any discarnate energy. This is why "dabbling in the occult" is dangerous. In this, as in all spiritual matters, Christians seek the wisdom and discernment of Christ.

The word "demon" comes from the Greek *daimon*, which means malignant spirit or evil angel. In the New Testament, demons are seen as part of the Devil's opposition to God's saving grace by doing harm to humans. Jesus used God's power to limit and repel demons in a number of instances:

Matthew 8:28-34   Two Gadarene demoniacs
Matthew 9:32-33   A mute, demon-possessed man
Matthew 17:14-18   A boy with a demon
Mark 1:23-26   A man in the synagogue with an unclean spirit

During the Middle Ages and the Reformation, it was assumed that demons swarmed about everywhere, availing themselves of every opportunity to do harm to humans, to spite God. They caused disease, accidents, madness, and death; they hurt animals, and caused natural disasters. Their greatest satisfaction was corrupting the human soul. Demons watched every thought, and waited for any openness of the mind to sin, that they might rush in.

Even in that mentality, however, it was recognized that God would not al-low demons to tempt beyond our ability to resist, and they could be dispersed at any time by calling upon God's name and God's power.

These beliefs prevailed from the 14th to the 17th century. They fueled the excesses of witch hunting. In reaction to these excesses, and with the growth of rationalism, liberalism, and the scientific approach, activities previously blamed on the Devil and demons began to be attributed to natural causes and psycho-logical processes.

Since the 1930s, however, certain evangelical and charismatic churches and groups have renewed attention to the presence and activity of the Devil. Today not only theological conservatives but many people both within and without the church are acknowledging the push and pull of opposing forces in their lives. Paul spoke of his own experience of inner conflict:

> *I do not do the good I want, but the evil I do not want is what I do.*
> (Romans 7:19)

As we discover more about the unconscious, we are made aware of the energies that operate in the personal and collective unconscious and their impact on us. In the psychology of C. G. Jung, the awareness and integration of opposites is a necessary step in becoming a fully conscious individual. These opposites within the psyche are variously identified: masculine and feminine, light and dark-ness, good and evil. Bringing awareness of these into the conscious mind is considered part of our human maturing. We come to greater understanding of ourselves, and of the powers that work within us.

Richard Foster says in *Coming Home: A Prayer Journal,*

> *When in honesty we accept the evil that is in us as*
> *part of the truth about ourselves and offer that truth up to God,*
> *we are in a mysterious way nourished.*
> *Even the truth about our shadow side sets us free.*

Exorcising Demons

Scott Peck, in his book *People of the Lie,* insists there can be more at work than a normal integrative process. He tells of psychological/spiritual work with persons oppressed and possessed. There is no doubt in his mind that demonic powers can and do influence and sometimes infiltrate the life of human persons.

In thinking about this book, the question arose for us: "Can we write a book on Christian Healing and not include a discussion of prayer for exorcism?" Although Christian healing or prayer teams are not likely to need to perform exorcisms, nor feel equipped to do so, we do need to be informed about them.

Occasionally in healing and prayer ministry, we may see manifestations that appear to us to be demonic. But we must not look for demons or "unclean spirits" where there are none! Addictive and compulsive behaviors are not in themselves evidence of an infiltrating spirit. Such untreated and chronic conditions may leave a person vulnerable to demonic intrusion, but we should not assume demonic possession. However, if a person is obsessed by debilitating fears or behavior that neither psychological therapy nor strong prayer can release, then the possibility of a terrorizing spirit may need to be considered.

Scott Peck explains that genuine Satanic possession is very rare, but can happen. In such cases he advises that such prayer be undertaken only by the power of the Christ and the gifts of the Spirit, and only by a team of persons who are mature in faith, experienced in prayer, and prepared by knowledge and skill.

Wayne had an unusual experience where congregational healing was needed. A spirit of bitterness had, over a long time, infiltrated the church, destroying peace, causing hurt and dissension among the people, and even causing some to depart. The normal methods of dealing with internal dissension didn't work. Having pondered and prayed about this situation over a whole summer's holiday, Wayne returned in the fall feeling urged to take some spiritual action. He prepared the congregation by preaching on Jesus' exorcisms, and lovingly shared with them his discernment of the spirit in their midst. At the close of the sermon, he stepped to the center of the chancel, pointed into the nave above and beyond the people's heads, named the spiritual energy, "Bitterness," and banished it in the name of Christ. Then, in a natural manner, he proceeded with the balance of the service.

From that day on, the mood and tone of meetings were different. So were people's conversations. Whenever even a hint of bitterness appeared, someone would say, "We don't allow that around here anymore!" The people took authority over the spirit of bitterness themselves because of the Sunday morning experience.

Through such sources, there has come a revival of awareness of the existence of evil powers in the universe, the "principalities and powers" against which we wrestle.

But we should not become obsessed by their powers. Aldous Huxley observed that the effects which follow too constant and intense a concentration upon evil are always disastrous. By having our focus primarily on evil, he said, we tend "to create occasions for evil to manifest," no matter how excellent our intentions. It is wisdom, therefore, to keep our eyes, our thoughts and our hearts tuned to that which is true, pure, excellent and worthy of praise, as Paul instructed the Philippians (chapter 4:8). By focusing on God and the good in the world, by lifting up the name of Jesus, by raising our voices in praise, we do our part in keeping our personal energies clean, clear, and strong, and our spirits invulnerable.

Angels

But if there are demons, there are also angels.

The Bible teaches us that the energies in the spiritual dimension include the created beings of light called angels. These beings come into our lives in various ways: as persons, in visions or dreams, in a felt presence, in a voice or in singing, or as inspiration that comes to the mind or through the intuition.

And they come into our lives unexpectedly.

Bonnie was 17, living in Kenora, Ontario. In 1971, on March break, she was traveling by bus to Thunder Bay. With her friend, Suzanne, she boarded the bus at midnight, with a bucket of fried chicken to nourish them on the journey. Settling in the second last seat, she noticed a young man in the last seat. He had dark blonde shoulder length hair, and his eyes, she says, "were an endless blue." She offered him a piece of chicken, to which he responded softly, "No thank you. I don't eat meat; I'm a vegetarian. But I appreciate your kindness."

Soon Suzanne was asleep, but Bonnie remained restless. She sneaked a glance at their vegetarian neighbor. He looked ordinary enough, dressed in jeans, a heavy wool sweater, and a dark green parka that he had tossed onto the seat next to him.

He caught her gaze. "Do you feel like talking?" he asked.

"Sure," she replied. "I've never met a vegetarian before."

They laughed together. Bonnie moved to sit next to him, and the two began a conversation that lasted all night.

They talked philosophy, religion, the war in Vietnam, their experiences of the world, and Bonnie's struggles with Christianity – the contradiction between gospel and church as institution. Bonnie says,

*He listened and didn't attempt to correct or shush me. He listened
intently and then asked me what I could do. How could I make a
difference in this world? Instead of rejecting Christianity, why
didn't I practice it in the way I felt in my heart was right for me? I
recall shaking my head in amazement. We laughed softly together,
and I remember the peacefulness and joy I felt that night. It was
grace, a freedom I had never experienced before.*

As morning approached, Suzanne joined them. The young man said his name
was Wes. And as the lights of Thunder Bay glowed in the distance, Bonnie
recalls feeling a sense of wonder:

*My body was tingling. I felt as if I had spent the night suspended
in the sky, dancing with the northern lights.
Everything around me seemed to glow,
even the tired snow packed on the curbs surrounding our bus.*

*I don't actually remember saying goodbye to our new friend.
I do recall him touching my long brown hair and saying,
"Go in peace."*

*"Thank you," was all I replied. I then kneeled down to retrieve our
bulging knapsacks and when I stood up he was gone.*

"What happened last night?" Suzanne asked.

*"I'm not sure," I replied. "But I know I feel different;
something inside of me has changed." I felt as if I had experienced
another dimension, one that reached beyond words.
I was also radiating with an energy that felt new and exciting.
I made an important decision. I decided to follow my heart.
I stopped eating meat. I felt as if in some way I had experienced a
resurrection. Twenty-six years later, I am still celebrating the
sacredness in all living beings. I am still a vegetarian.
Occasionally I close my eyes
and visualize Wes standing next to me.
He touched something in me that night that was precious.*

My life during these past number of years
hasn't always been peaceful.
Yet through it all, I have remembered his words,
"Go in peace." I have tried to honor his blessing.
As I reflect back on that wonder-filled night, I know in my heart
that Wes was a messenger sent from God.
Wes was, and probably still is, an angel.
His presence in my life that night was a miracle.

The Presence of Angels

The word "angel" comes from the Greek *angelos* meaning "messenger." Angels are God's messengers – beings who do God's bidding. Hebrews 1:14 refers to "angels in the divine service." They never draw attention to themselves, but work to promote God's plans and bring about God's highest good for us. They are mentioned directly or indirectly nearly 300 times in the Bible.

Genesis 16:7	Hagar and the angel
Genesis 32:2	Jacob meets two angels
Exodus 3:2	Moses and the burning bush
Numbers 20:16	Exodus from Egypt
Judges 6:11-12	Gideon and the angel
1 Kings 19:5	Elijah under the broom tree
Daniel 3:25	An angel in the fire
Matthew 1:20	Joseph and angel in a dream
Luke 1:13	Angel and Zechariah
Luke 1:26	Announcement to Mary
Luke 2:9-10	Shepherds and angel
Matthew 4:11	Jesus in the wilderness
Luke 22:43	Jesus on Mount of Olives
Luke 16:22	Story of the poor man Lazarus
Matthew 28:2,5	Angels at resurrection
Acts 8:26	Philip and the angel
Acts 12:7-9	Peter's release from prison
Acts 27:23-24	Paul in the storm
Revelation 1:1	Revelation of John

Many healers today have an awareness of being helped from beyond themselves. Some feel another hand or hands placed over their own when laying on hands for healing. Or their own hands are picked up, moved, and placed on another without conscious volition.

Rochelle speaks of her own experience:

> *We were about to begin the Sacred Chakra Spread*
> *(described in Appendix B) when Lisa arrived late*
> *from a memorial service. She described how difficult the service*
> *had been, and she talked about the pain in her heart.*
> *She felt the weight of what she was carrying as physically painful.*

In the debriefing that followed, Lisa herself told this story:

> *I really wondered what they [the two people doing the healing*
> *work] were doing. I knew that the technique was to come to an*
> *end with their hands on my heart, and yet from the beginning I*
> *felt hands on my chest.*
> *I then realized that my partners were doing the technique in the*
> *correct sequence. These hands were the hands of an angel. I could*
> *see this angel hold my heart in her hands, and I could see all the*
> *darkness, all the pain being transformed. The light was pouring*
> *from the angel's hands, and my heart was being mended. The*
> *pain is now gone. I feel as though a great weight has just been*
> *lifted. I feel completely different.*

It is common in healing workshops, while people are receiving, to experience the presence of angels – spiritual helpers sent by God to assist. Some people will actually see their presence while receiving the healing. Others will simply feel extra hands on their bodies, and describe the sensation of a very loving presence. They will say they knew they were being held with loving hands.

A Catholic priest in one of Rochelle's workshops felt the extra set of hands, and opened his eyes to see who was there. Not seeing anyone, he trusted the physical sensation, relaxed, and later reported to the class that these were the hands of his angels.

Avoiding Negative Influences

We cannot always be certain that our prayers align perfectly with God's will, but these things we can do:

1. Ask ourselves, "Is this prayer truly loving? Is it something Jesus would have prayed?"
2. Accept the shadow side of our own personalities, and cooperate with God in the transformation and integration of our conscious awareness.
3. Be assured that the Holy Spirit will purify our prayers, when our intent is love.
4. Remember to put on "the whole armor of God" day by day.
5. Remember the words of Peter:

> *Have unity of spirit, sympathy, love for one another, a tender*
> *heart, and a humble mind. Do not repay evil for evil or abuse*
> *for abuse; but, on the contrary, repay with a blessing. It is*
> *for this that you were called – that you might inherit a blessing.*
> (1 Peter 3:8-9)

The Spindrift experiments seem to demonstrate the presence of a "loving intelligence" which directs prayer where and how it is most needed. These are not isolated discoveries.
Wayne Irwin *identifies a host of other scientific and laboratory experiments which push our understanding even further.*

10

The Loving Intelligence Of the Universe

The nature of the universe seems to be rooted in pattern, which can be thought of as "order" or "goodness." It also is beset with deviations from pattern, which might be thought of as "disorder" or "evil." The fact that a person praying can not visualize the particulars of what is needed for healing is apparently of no more importance to the outcome than not knowing how toenails grow or why falling bread always lands butter-side down. The loving intelligence apparently does not depend upon the one praying having this knowledge.

The pervasiveness of this loving intelligence goes even further. Mind and matter appear to be even more closely linked than experimental evidence has previously shown. Robert Jahn, with the Princeton Engineering Anomalies Research (PEAR) program, suggests that every characteristic of matter – its size, its shape, its dimensions, and its structure – appears to arise completely from the spiritual domain, from information being sourced by this loving intelligence.

The apostle John, 19 centuries ago, wrote,

In the beginning was the Word…All things came into being through him, and without him not one thing came into being.
(John 1:1, 3)

Physicist David Bohm invites us to think of mind and body as an indivisible entity like a bar magnet, the mind like the North pole and the body like the

South. Nowhere can one cut the magnet to have North in one hand and South in another. No matter how it is divided, each fragment of that magnet will still have both North and South poles.

In the same way, mind and body are linked, as are the individual and the entity we have called "the loving intelligence."

Daniel Benor comments that logic would suggest that when a healer engages in prayer for a person with infection or cancer, without reference to the divine will – that is, with focused intention towards a particular outcome –one might expect there to be some unwelcome side effects. None have ever been reported. Sometimes, Benor notes, the benefits show up in areas of the patient's being that were not targeted. When this happens, it can be now be apparently understood in terms of the mixing of goal-directed and identity-directed prayer.

Stimulating the Activity of Enzymes

The laying on of hands with prayer has been shown to accelerate the activity of enzymes in the laboratory. In 1972, Justa Smith, a former Roman Catholic religious and a research scientist, performed some experimental work with Hungarian healer Oskar Estebany. She had him lay his hands on a stoppered glass flask containing the enzyme trypsin for a period of 75 minutes. Portions of the solution were removed for testing every 15 minutes. The longer Estebany prayed for the enzymes, the greater was their activity.

The results of such tests suggest that healing prayer with the laying on of hands may assist recuperation from illness by contributing to the hormonal balance. However, experimentation on another occasion, when Estebany was not feeling well, made it evident that his personal state of mind and body made a significant difference to the effectiveness of his prayer.

This supports the view that preparation is essential for a healing prayer team, and that each person on the team should be in a state of personal peace before entering into intentional involvement in prayer for the condition of another. Other work by Glen Rein and Rollin McCraty in California has demonstrated that the brain waves of a person being prayed for will actually entrain – come into the same rhythm – with those of the person praying, provided the heart connection is in place.

The Effect of Negative Attitudes

Norman Cousins, an initiator of the new medical field of psycho-neuro-immunology, has reported how negative attitudes in the patient or the surrounding family or friends can contribute to worsening conditions, in the patient or among members of the caring group. He himself prolonged his life by the shift in his emotional state that resulted from learning to laugh. And in *Head First: The Biology of Hope,* he tells of an encounter with a patient at Encino Hospital in California. The patient was a judge in the terminal stage of cancer, whose mood was understandably bleak. Throughout his life, he had been known for his positive outlook on life. Cousins was asked to see him because the judge's attitude was having a devastating effect upon his family.

Cousins developed rapport with him, and then told him of his research findings: that the attitude of a patient always had a profound effect upon the family. He told the judge that the health of his family members was being jeopardized by his negative attitude about his own impending death. Cousins reported that the judge, known for his courage and determinism, closed his eyes momentarily while he absorbed this information. Then he opened them, and uttered just two words: "I gotcha."

Two weeks later, Cousins learned that the judge had decisively changed his attitude. He had called for food. He had talked with his wife about problems that came up in tournament bridge games. He had resumed reading the newspaper, taking walks in the hospital corridor, and conversing with other patients. His doctor, who had expected that he would not survive the first weekend, was amazed. The judge survived several more weeks, not just prolonging his own life, but bolstering the lives of the others around him. His sense of purpose did not reverse the progress of the disease, but, Cousins said, it clearly enabled him to govern the particulars of his passing in a way that was consistent with his life.

People often understand this truth intuitively, without needing research documentation. One of my parishioners had a terminally ill wife. A number of "gloomy Gus" visitors had been around, all long faces and sorrow. The parishioner muttered to me: "I wish these crepe-hangers would stay home. She's still with us. She's not yet gone, and we want to enjoy the time together that we still have." The communal mindset was enveloping a patient in a cloud of hopelessness.

Negative mindsets are a hurdle that must be cleared by any healing prayer.

Preventative Benefits

Daniel Benor finds evidence healing prayer can even be preventative. Conditions such as influenza, bovine foot and mouth disease, and anticipated difficult childbirths may be beneficially moderated by advance use of healing methods. And the evidence gathered by epidemiologist and writer Jeffrey Levin, of published reports over the past 100 years, shows the benefits of regular religious practice to be statistically comparable to the benefits of stopping smoking. Perhaps those who cannot give up cigarettes could instead be encouraged to get themselves regularly into church!

The Effect of Expectations

G. K and A. M. Watkins reported on the selective wakening of one of a pair of anesthetized mice by the specific intention of the healer. Their work suggests that healing prayer can be measurably effective in reducing the negative affects of anesthesia during and after surgery.

In working with malarial mice, Gerry Solfvin found that when experimenters were not told which mice were designated to receive healing, the experimenter's own expectations produced a modest healing effect. This phenomenon, also noted by the Spindrift group, has been named "The Rosenthal Effect." The name comes from R. Rosenthal's 1978 study of the effect of the experimenter's beliefs on outcome. Rosenthal suggested that it might actually be possible for *any* hypothesis to be proven if an experimenter believed strongly enough in its truth. Herbert Benson's more recent tests, showing that the doctor's attitude toward the medicine being prescribed makes a difference, support Rosenthal's conclusions.

The Power of Suggestion

Dr. Henry K. Beecher of Massachusetts General Hospital conducted a study in 1961 on a type of cardiac surgery known as "internal mammary artery ligation," a procedure which ties off arteries that seem to divert blood unnecessarily away from the heart. Patients undergoing this surgery reported decided improvement; objective tests confirmed positive indications. However, the ligation did involve major surgery, with its inherent risks. Beecher chose to test the so-called "placebo effect" by dividing his patients into two groups. One group underwent the complete treatment. The other group received only a skin wound, instead of the full surgical process they expected. But, when they came out of anesthesia, both would look exactly the same.

Amazingly, the patients who received only a skin wound improved at the same rate and to the same extent as the others. Their improvement was not just subjective; it registered even on their tests. Beecher's studies, in general, seemed to indicate a 30 percent success rate.

The placebo effect is credited with a known fact – people tend to get better at the same rate whether they see a doctor or simply make an appointment. Because critics were challenging Harvard researcher Herbert Benson's studies on the measurable benefits of meditation, and attributing them to the placebo effect, Benson launched his own studies. He found the placebo effect to be at least twice as powerful as previously understood.

Clearly, what people believe – about themselves and about their treatment – has a decided effect on their own healing.

The Effect of Visualization on Immune Systems

G. F. Solomon, another researcher, reported the results of studies where visualization enhanced the immune system. Some of these experiments were with AIDS or HIV patients, and some remarkable recoveries have been reported where traditional approaches had failed. Here again, the public media reflect the conventional wisdom that such an illness is "always fatal." But the truth is that even in 1981, when the disease was first defined, up to 8 percent were surviving. That number has been increasing ever since.

In related studies, Elmer and Alyce Green, founders of the Biological Feedback research program at the Menninger Foundation in Kansas, have shown that the patient's self-image and expectations are vitally important. Both factors, of course, are influenced by social views of AIDS.

The Greens have demonstrated even more profound changes in the patient's well-being if the person uses self-constructed imagery rather than the guided imagery provided by others. The participation of the patient in choosing his or her own visual symbolism clearly helps.

The Effect on Pain

Gloria writes of her experience with pain:

> *In July of 1996, my husband Allan began to have pain in the front muscle of his leg. He went to the chiropractor several times in a seven-week period. He did not receive any relief from the treatments. At this point, the pain was going to the back of his leg, and he was beginning to limp. He was unable to walk for any length of time. I had just learned Therapeutic Touch, and gave him a treatment on the full leg. He said afterwards that he felt very relaxed during the procedure, and that while my hands felt very hot to him, his leg had felt cold. Now, a year later, with no further treatment, he has never experienced pain again in his leg.*

Similarly, Jeanne Beth writes,

> *The pain started in September. It was concentrated in my left*
> *shoulder and radiated down my whole left arm. In November, my*
> *family physician referred me to a physiotherapist. I received*
> *treatments from January to April, and my shoulder and arm had*
> *improved, but certainly had not healed. Physio could do no more*
> *for me. Two weeks later, the pain had returned in full force.*
> *At a weekend prayer retreat, Flora and Wayne gave me a*
> *Therapeutic Touch treatment, as I was in considerable discomfort.*
> *During the process, the pain became extremely intense, but I did*
> *not tell them. When I arose after the treatment, the pain was gone.*
> *Within five minutes I felt something being released from my*
> *shoulder. My arm was totally healed, and has remained so for*
> *over two years since. I am a practitioner of TT now myself, and*
> *use it on family, friends and our pet.*

While healing is most often an extended process, often the first treatment of Healing Touch procedures will alleviate pain. This effect has actually been demonstrated in only two published studies: one printed in *Nursing Research* in 1986, involving the effects of Therapeutic Touch on tension headache pain; the other in *Subtle Energies* in 1991, reporting on the effects of "a bioenergy healing technique" on chronic pain. However, the *1978 Report of the Ernest Holmes Research Foundation* of Los Angeles indicates that pain is actually the most common symptom reported as being alleviated by healing work.

Other surveys of patients indicate that most feel that, in their experience, healing work is always beneficial, even when no objective evidence exists.

Doctoral work in the early 1970s by nursing research scientist Janet Quinn, (along with other more recent studies by Patricia Heidt, R. B. Fedoruk and B. S. Parkes) have shown definitively that healing work reduces anxiety. Clinical reports always seem to mention that when a healing treatment is used, the patients visibly relax. They often become flushed, and occasionally evidence drowsiness. Because of Quinn's pioneering experimental work and the large number of subsequent scientific dissertations on the subject, Therapeutic Touch is proving acceptable to the medical establishment, and is now officially appended to the policies and procedures of many hospitals across North America.

The Human Electromagnetic Field

Away back in 1882, A. P. Sinnett, the editor of *The Pioneer*, an English language newspaper of India, published a description of how student Tibetan monks developed their perception. Every temple had a dark room, with its north wall entirely covered with a highly polished sheet of metal, mainly copper. The student monk sat in front of the wall, on a three-legged bench placed on thick glass. A bar magnet was suspended over the student monk's head, without touching it. The student monk sat there alone, staring at the wall, meditating.

Inspired by this old report, Elmer Green in Kansas initiated a research project to measure human electromagnetic fields. He tested the difference between the electrical charge of a person at rest and a person at prayer. Green designed what he called a Copper Wall Laboratory, and began testing subjects.

He found that during meditation a build-up of electrical charge on the body occurred. This increase was more pronounced for persons trained in Non-Contact Therapeutic Touch (NCTT) than for ordinary meditators. When the body potential of the NCTT persons was measured during treatment sessions, brief voltage surges were recorded at the moment of their focusing. With regular meditators, no surge registered more than 4 volts. But with trained NCTT meditators, a burst of electrical activity ranged from 4 up to 221 volts! The average was 8.3 volts, with the duration of the surge averaging 3.6 seconds.

Green and his colleagues concluded that NCTT therapists had a different "bioenergy-handling capability" from untrained persons. Their intention to heal seemed to be related to the strength of the electrical surges. He also concluded that his tests gave evidence of a normally undeveloped capability within the human system.

The phenomenon seemed related to the ancient concept of the "vital energy of the body." Almost every culture has such a concept, though each culture gives it a different name. The Chinese called it *Qi* (pronounced "chee"). Indian science named it *prana*. Long ago, Hippocrates referred to it as *vis medicatrix naturae* (the natural energy of health). Kabbalists called it "astral light." Ambrose and Olga Worrall referred to it as "para-electricity." Wilhelm Reich termed it "orgone energy." Other names have been *pneuma* or "spirit" (Pythagoras), "life beams" (Robert Fludd), "pre-physical energy" (George de la Warr), and "DC fields" (Robert Becker).

Qi Can Enter From External Sources

David Eisenberg went to the People's Republic of China in 1982 with a medical delegation to study Qi. He described their experiences in *Encounters with Qi*. The group included Herbert Benson, of Harvard. Benson agreed to participate in a demonstration, to receive "external Qi" from a Dr. Zhou, a Qi Gong master on the faculty of the Shanghai First Medical College.

Benson stood in the middle of the room with his eyes closed, his hands at his side, his head slightly bowed, and entered into his own relaxation exercise. From about ten feet away, Dr. Zhou aimed his arms at the visiting doctor. Benson began swaying from side to side, to the point of almost losing his balance, of having to shift his feet. Then his hips began to twist, first to the right, then to the left. He jerkily turned through 180 degrees. At this point Dr. Zhou stepped forward and placed his right hand on Benson's neck. He was, in his word, "removing excess Qi." Benson subsequently insisted that he had initiated all of the movements himself, to resist Dr. Zhou's actions. He was not convinced that Zhou could actually move him against his will. Nevertheless, he did concede that he had definitely experienced a sensation of physical pressure coming from the Qi master, even though he was standing ten feet away. In that sense, even the ever-scientific Benson confirmed the power of Qi. The only question was whether it had caused his movements directly or indirectly.

Experiments with Love

In the early decades of the 20th century, the investigation of love was excluded from scientific study. As an emotion, it fell outside the interests of science at the time. But love is now recognized to have effects, whether love is understood as universal energy, or simply as a personal, subjective experience with psychological and social roots.

Many of these effects are now being studied. Three research scientists working at the HeartMath Institute in California devised a project to measure "love." They set about measuring the effect of one persons's intentional love on the physiology of another. William Gough, Rollin McCraty, and Glen Rein presented their findings in 1994 at the annual conference of the International Society for the Study of Subtle Energy and Energy Medicine (ISSSEEM). For their particular study, Gough, McCraty, and Rein defined love as "the benevolent concern for the well-being of others expressed in a true, sincere, feeling state." Researcher Gough, who with Robert Shacklett had developed the working model of reality based on the ideas of Cambridge mathematician Roger Penrose, stated his conviction that this work was an aspect of a new "science of connectiveness," within which, he suggested, "love" is the key organizing principle.

Faster than the Speed of Light

In the mid-1960s, John Bell, an Irish physicist working in Geneva, had addressed this connectiveness. He proposed an experiment, involving two photons emitted by an atom simultaneously in two directions. By definition of quantum physics, he noted, the photons would be "polarized" – that is, they would be spinning or pointing in different directions. Discovering the spin of one photon would immediately determine the spin of the other. However, in the quantum world, everything is uncertain until it is observed. And furthermore, the act of observing determines the findings. Their state, therefore, would be indeterminate until someone actually took the first measurement. Meanwhile, the photons, moving at the speed of light, could theoretically have traveled virtually across the universe from each other. But the act of measuring and thus determining the spin of one would force the other one to assume the opposite spin direction. The communication between the two would thus have to be faster than the speed of light. It would be instantaneous. The information would have to travel at infinite speed.

The idea of it all came to be known as Bell's Theorem.

Gough, McCraty, and Rein suspected that the bond of love between two human beings was actually the same phenomenon at the human level as Bell's Theorem at the quantum level. For the heart connection, the associational link, neither distance nor time holds any meaning. They suggested, therefore, that the heart connection is transcendent, that love is the channel for instructions from some higher level entering our three-dimensional reality.

In Spindrift terms, Gough, McCraty and Rein were presenting additional evidence of the involvement of a "loving intelligence."

The three California scientists proposed that deep feelings of love may affect the templates or patterns that inform the development of our bodies and that connect us to the spiritual ordering principle. This connection, they suggested, affects physiological balance. By invoking it, health may be restored in any or every system of the body, provided that the individual recipient removes any self-imposed "constraints." The persons being treated – the recipients – must intentionally open themselves, intentionally bring their system into a state of readiness to receive the spiritual information that will resonate with the perfect patterns of the divine will.

At the ISSSEEM conference, Gough, McCraty, and Rein presented their evidence as to how this resonance results in scientifically measurable changes. In a study of AIDS/HIV persons, they found that changes in attitude towards an appreciative loving state correlated with changes in brain waves, which, in turn, correlated with changes in the hormonal and immune responses of the body. In other words, they offered scientific evidence of the healing power of love!

The Measurable Effects of Love

Theirs is not the only scientific test of the power of love. William Braud, a Senior Research Associate at the Mind Science Foundation in Texas, did experiments in which people donated a small quantity of their own blood. Their human red blood cells were put into a salt solution that would cause them to rupture. The donors were then asked to protect their own blood cells in the test tubes, by loving them, by visualizing them as happy, healthy cells, and by imagining the membranes of their blood cells being resilient, warding off the chemical pressure that would otherwise kill them.

Certain people were indeed able to protect and change the rate at which their red blood cells were dying, compared to a control group. He also found they could protect the cells of another person, although as expected that effect was not as robust as when they focused on their own cells.

Other work by McCraty and Rein supports this finding. They demonstrated, in their laboratory, that a loving heart can even influence the winding and the unwinding of the DNA (deoxyribonucleic acid, the genetic material) within a single cell. This is utterly astounding. It indicates that we may have the ability to affect not only the behavior of another person through clear mental intention, but we can also influence the behavior of individual cells and even the organizing elements within those cells.

Healing Starts from the Heart

They report that, apart from everything else that it does, the heart functions as a master electrical oscillator. It radiates frequencies which promote the health and vitality of the entire human system. The ability we are now shown to possess, to direct an intention to a specific DNA molecule, indicates that the energy field associated with the state of deep love can respond to very explicit intentions. It is not just something nebulous and vague, without order.

Their findings offer the first published experimental evidence showing that the sustained loving state can produce physiological effects in the building blocks of life itself. Healing starts from the heart!

McCraty, with Mike Atkinson and William Tiller of Stanford University, conducted another related study. They used a registered focusing technique developed at the HeartMath Institute called "Freeze-Frame." In this method of meditation, persons focus solely on the heart area of their bodies. They intentionally generate a feeling of appreciation for someone or something else, maintaining this feeling for a period of time.

Using traditional means of measuring heart rate variability, McCraty, Atkinson, and Tiller observed that this technique brought about an automatic enhancement of the meditating person's autonomic nervous system. In other words, this meditative practice led to improved self-management of the mental and emotional states that affect the whole body, including the brain. Practitioners of these heart-focus techniques also reported increased intuitive awareness, and a more efficient decision-making capability. McCraty concluded from this that consciousness is clearly not limited to the brain/mind interface. The heart is definitely involved.

These experiments extend our understanding of the new and currently popular psycho-neuro-immunology model which considers only the effects of brain/mind on the immune system. They indicate that the heart regulates the ability of the brain/mind to affect the body. Even loving one's dog or cat or teddy bear, in other words, is measurably beneficial to one's health. It is possible that a sustained loving state enhances immunity by indeed acting directly on our DNA. This new understanding of the role of the heart, they suggest, opens up a brand new area of disciplined scientific investigation. They call it "cardio-neuro-immunology."

Further studies have examined the attitude or intention of the persons doing healing prayer. They have shown that sincere feelings of appreciation, love, and care do enhance the inner biological systems of the one doing the praying. This is significant, because the heart generates the strongest electromagnetic field produced by the body, a field that can be measured a number of feet away with SQUID-based magnetometers and sensitive electrostatic detectors. ("SQUID" is an acronym for "superconducting quantum interference device" – *very* high tech!)

The Effect of Love on Inanimate Objects

Beverly Rubik, of Temple University, conducted another experiment using a random event generator device. Operator Terry Ross attempted to influence the random output of the machine.

Rubik observed from preliminary feedback that Ross was generating statistically insignificant scores from the very beginning. So she asked him about his attitude toward the device. He replied that he disliked it. She asked him then whether there was any way that he might be able to change his attitude toward it. Ross thought for a moment, and then with a big grin he gathered it up in his arms and began to cuddle the device as though it were a puppy.

In the next run he achieved a positive score that was over three standard deviations above the mean value. In other words, the measurable effect of love on the machine's output was astonishing.

Among Rubik's conclusions about what she calls "psi phenomena" – the manifestation of measurable healing benefit – is her considered opinion that this effect arises from the deepest and most intimate realms of our being. She says that future research in this area must include not only the psychological but also the spiritual domain, to accommodate the full depth and breadth of human experience.

She also echoes a conclusion from quantum physics. The integrity, authenticity, and personal commitment of the scientist doing the research, says Rubik, truly affects the outcome. The observer is very much a part of the observed.

The Effect of Skepticism and Depression

Bernard Grad, of McGill University, working with Remi Cadoret and G. I. Paul of the University of Manitoba, noted something similar in earlier studies. They measured how quickly wounds healed in mice held by healer Oskar Estebany, compared with a control group. But they also observed mice held in the same way by skeptical medical students healed consistently *slower* than the control group. Skepticism actually inhibited normal healing.

In a related study, Grad had a man with a psychotic depression participate as a healer. As in other experiments of this type, this man laid his hands on a sealed bottle containing water that would be used on the plants. This depressed man's efforts produced the worst results of all, compared with the others.

These findings have implications for our social relationships. In a study of persons who died during 1974, Judith and Robert Shellenberger reported that of all the variables considered, social network had the highest correlation with health and longevity. Close relationships with spouse, family, and friends had more significant health benefits than even church and social organization membership. (And church association, as Jeffrey Levin found, has as much effect on health as non-smoking!) Persons with many close social ties, the Shellenbergers asserted, have a lower risk of early death than those with few social ties. And even persons with unhealthy lifestyle behaviors, if they have close social ties, tend to live longer than persons with healthy behaviors who lack those close social ties.

Resistance to Being Loved

Leonard Laskow, in his book *Healing with Love*, states that the source of most of our maladies is our inability to love ourselves or to open ourselves to receive love from others. When illness arises, we generally focus on treating symptoms. But we could instead go to the source of the disorder and make changes there.

He considers the common cold as an example. Recent studies have suggested that colds are "caused" by a virus. Other studies show that even when we have no cold, we still harbor the virus. So our immune system is definitely involved. We also know that stress is a major factor affecting the immune system. And new studies hint that fear of losing control lies at the root of most stress.

So the question arises: Do we get colds partly because we are unwilling to trust the divine love? Because we close ourselves to its expression in the love of others?

The Sources of Illness

The primary source for any illness, says Laskow, is our perceptions and interpretations. Our mental, emotional, or physical well-being is influenced by the meaning that we attach to what is going on around us. A second level, he says, is our sense of worthiness. Persons who believe the worst about themselves close themselves off from restorative love. A third level, he suggests, has to do with whether or not we take an active role in our own well-being, or whether we passively surrender our opportunity and freedom to participate.

And the fourth level, Laskow continues, depends upon being tuned out or tuned in to the loving intention of God. In this, he mirrors the conclusions of Victor Frankl, in his classic *Man's Search for Meaning*. In the book, Frankl explored why he and some others survived the horrors of the Auschwitz concentration camp during the Holocaust, while others did not. His studies initiated the renowned psychiatric therapeutic procedure based on meaning, now known as "logotherapy."

Carl Simonton and Stephanie Matthews-Simonton have had significant success in working with cancer patients. They are perhaps best known for encouraging patients to use creative and constructive imagery to combat their illness.

The Simontons suggest that the biggest single factor predisposing a person to cancer is grief – the loss of a serious love. This commonly occurs between 6 to 18 months prior to diagnosis. The loss, they say, whether it is real or imagined, must be very significant.

Even more important than the actual loss, they say, is the emotional response of the person suffering it. The loss has to produce a feeling of helplessness and hopelessness. It becomes more than a simple loss. It becomes a symbol for the person's life. That person begins to physically die.

Healing as a Matter of the Heart

This is but a sampling of the investigative work currently examining what can be known about healing from the heart. It indicates that all healing is unquestionably a matter, first and foremost, of the heart. As Einstein put it: "Body and soul are not two different things, but only two ways of perceiving the same thing."

Robert Jahn said it in a different way: "What consciousness experiences, it attempts to comprehend. To comprehend, it must order. To order, it must name, and in the naming, it creates its experience."

"Naming" is an ancient and honorable tradition. In the words of Genesis 2:19:

Out of the ground the LORD God formed every animal of the field
and every bird of the air, and brought them to the man to see
what he would call them; and whatever the man called every
living creature, that was its name.

As it is for mice and soybeans, for rye seed and for enzymes, so it must be for heart, for love, for consciousness, and for life itself.

*Prayer works. It can be either private, or public. Services of public prayer invite the entire congregation or faith community to be involved. **Flora Litt** describes some of the preparation and action for healing prayer services.*

11

Involving the Community of Faith

Healing has always been a major purpose and intention of the church. In *The Uncommon Touch*, Tom Harpur, popular Canadian religion and ethics writer, says that a reading of the Book of Acts quickly reveals the difference between lackluster mainline churches today and the vibrant, energy-filled church of apostolic times. According to Acts, Harpur observes, healing is not "some peripheral activity for fanatics, sectarians or mystics." Rather, healing lies at the heart of the mandate of the Christian community.

We are created with a need to worship. Since we are also created to live in community, it follows that we are drawn by our nature to communal worship. Since Neanderthal humans first gathered bear skulls in a cave – the earliest known activity of spiritual, archetypal significance – and down through the ages, religious ritual has never ceased. Even when driven underground by persecution, Christians still found ways to meet and worship together.

Isolation is death. Community is life – or is intended to be! And so the church today, a carrier of the Word of abundant life, is called to care for the wellness and health not only of its members, but through these to care for the wider community of the world.

True caring is total. And total caring includes body, mind, spirit, emotions, and relationships. This is the healing ministry of the community. In corporate ritual activity, we celebrate God's goodness and gifts more completely than we can alone.

It's true that Jesus had a private, "lonely hillside" prayer life, but he also assumed corporate praise and prayer to be the norm for his spiritual activity.

> *When he came to Nazareth, where he had been brought up, he*
> *went to the synagogue on the Sabbath day, as was his custom.*
> (Luke 4:16)

The ritual practices of synagogue and temple framed his days. There he questioned, challenged, read, taught, and prayed. And in response to his disciples' request to teach them to pray, he began with a collective invocation: *"Our Father...".* By healing the man with the unclean spirit in the synagogue in Capernaum, he brought healing right into the center of the communal ritual (Mark 1:21-27).

Similarly, Acts 2:42-47 describes the life of the believers after Jesus was with them only in spirit. They spent much time together in the temple, and broke bread from house to house. They stayed close together, sharing their common story, caring for one another, and being strengthened for their ministry. Because they were built up in faith and in the Spirit, they were used by God wherever they were. So on their way to the temple at the hour of prayer, Peter healed a crippled beggar (Acts 3:1-9).

Corporate ritual activity is meant to empower the healed to be healers.

Laity and Clergy Together

I remember my childhood in The United Church of Canada. The elders of the church were spiritual leaders. They held positions of responsibility in the church; they cared for the well-being of the members of the flock assigned to them. In home visiting, as well as in church, they spoke openly and earnestly of their commitment to Jesus Christ, and comfortably conversed of spiritual matters. They always prayed with the family and knew each member well.

But over the years, more and more, discussion of spiritual matters was left to the pastor. Elders seemed less comfortable speaking of faith issues or praying. In many Protestant churches, educating and equipping lay people for spiritual healing or prayer ministry took second place to the study of issues and social action. Like the rest of our society, we in these churches tended to live mostly in our heads as we wrestled with issues that concern worship, baptism, inclusivity, and the nature of mission in the world. This may have been a needed corrective for the emotional pietism of our Methodist ancestors, for example, but it was also a loss.

Today, both financial necessity and a renewed focus on lay ministry means that more churches have Pastoral Care teams to assist clergy in caring for the community of faith. But many lay persons, although they understand that all Christians are called to ministry in the name of Jesus, may not feel adequate to the task.

So in any discussion of and planning for the beginning and maintaining of a healing ministry within the congregation or parish, both clergy and laity must be involved from the beginning, and throughout. This commitment gives clergy the opportunity to participate with lay persons in studying together the biblical and historical background of healing, and to share in deep discussions about what we as Christians believe about God, Jesus Christ, the Holy Spirit, prayer, and healing for the whole person. And it gives lay persons the opportunity to clarify their beliefs and deepen their faith as they reflect on their own experience, and on God's healing presence and activity in their lives, the church, and the world.

Preparing for a Healing Ministry

From my experience in working with parishes and congregations, I see a number of steps in moving towards an intentional healing ministry.

Building Some Familiarity with the Concept

The initial interest in a healing ministry in the local congregation/parish may come from an Order of Ministry person or a lay person. Someone may learn that a nearby church of any denomination has a healing ministry. A lay person or persons may attend a service with the clergy, for the shared experience and discussion afterwards. Or the initiative may come from a church member who has done some bioenergy work, who has experienced the laying on of hands in a secular setting through a Healing Touch, Therapeutic Touch, Reiki, or other therapeutic healing practice. Many lay persons and some clergy have either experienced such an energy-based healing, or have become practitioners or teachers themselves. Others may have seen something on television, or read about it, or know someone who does bioenergy work.

Opening the Subject for the Congregation or Parish

Having become aware of this interest and need, an opportunity for informal conversation or study/discussion opportunity should be offered. This should happen with authorization from the appropriate church body – Session, Council, Christian Development or Education Committee. It is important that, if and when a congregation/parish is ready to offer a healing ministry, it is seen both inside and outside the church as part of the ministry of the whole congregation/parish. A healing ministry cannot develop and maintain itself in a healthy way if it is not, in some measure, understood and supported by the whole community of faith.

Allowing the Spirit to Lead

Following this initial discussion and study, the next step(s) will no doubt be evident. But here are some ideas for consideration:

1. After the initial gathering and discussion, perhaps "let it lie" for a time. Let the idea of a healing ministry make its way informally into people's minds and hearts. Encourage people to seek various experiences of healing ministries in order to gain perspective.

2. Invite lay persons more frequently to accompany the clergy or other trained visitors to hospitals, homes of the sick, or nursing homes to hear and see prayer ministry in action, perhaps with communion, anointing, or the laying on of hands.

3. Begin a prayer group or a prayer chain, if the congregation/parish does not already have one. Often persons from a prayer group, where they have become comfortable hearing and eventually speaking prayer in an intimate setting, become part of the healing ministry. As the healing ministry develops in a more formal way, the prayer group is an essential support for the healing/prayer team. But remember that a prayer group or chain is not a means to an end – it is not just a way of leading people into a healing ministry. Prayer has its own worth, even if many members will never be at ease in "up front" healing ministry.

4. Place articles on healing in the church newsletter from time to time, and purchase some books for the church library.

5. Host a healing service. Invite a guest preacher and a healing team from another congregation/parish to come for the anointing, laying on of hands, and prayer ministry. This lets local congregational/parish members experience a healing service within their own setting and denomination.

6. Begin a more formal study program to prepare individuals for healing/prayer ministry. It should be open to all who wish to attend, with the clear understanding that not every person may feel called to become a member of a healing ministry team. This too should happen under the oversight of the Board of the congregation/parish.

Qualities of Healing Team Members

Healing team members do not need exceptional qualities, in my opinion. Indeed, exceptional qualities may be a deterrent. I suggest that they may be ordinary Christians who:

- Feel called by God to share in the healing ministry of Jesus Christ through the church.
- Have considerable clarity about their own beliefs, and a strong faith.
- Have experienced the grace of God in their own life.
- Love God with passion, and other people from a compassionate heart.
- Have a personal prayer life, and are at ease praying with others (experience in a team will increase the comfort level).
- Practice Christian meditation with regularity. (This not only grounds the personal life in Christ, but enables the deep centeredness and focused concentration necessary in healing work.)
- Are open and committed to ongoing spiritual growth, learning, and development of skills related to healing ministry.

Establishing a Support Group

In addition to the foreground ministry of prayer and healing, many tasks need to be done in the background. Persons are needed for publicity, preparing the Table and elements (this is best done by other than Healing/Prayer Team members), welcoming, ushering, taking up the offering, music, refreshments, and cleanup. There may be members of the congregation/parish who really care about and support the healing ministry and are only too willing to help in these ways, but do not feel called to the laying on of hands with prayer. Every contribution is important and part of the whole ministry. It is best to have one person as contact and organizer of this group.

Training the Teams

Training is essential to ensure that members do not disrupt a service by not knowing what to do, or where to be, and when. Not because a healing ministry must look polished and slick. But it should be orderly and calm, comfortable and comforting for those who come. As Paul said to the Corinthian church,

All things should be done decently and in order.
(1 Corinthians 14:40)

Paul did not say "rigidly" or "inflexibly." His intention was to give the Spirit freedom in the community while avoiding chaos.

Conclusion of Training

When training ends, all participants should be invited to decide whether or not they feel called to be part of a healing/prayer team, and whether they feel ready to begin.

A leader of the team needs to be identified and responsibilities laid out as follows:

1. To keep in touch with the Team members, and to be available to discuss concerns with them.
2. To be responsible for arranging partners for services, and for making any appointments for personal ministry that are needed.
3. To stay in close communication, on behalf of the team, with the clergy.
4. To call regular meetings of the healing/prayer team for prayer, sharing, reflection, and ongoing learning.
5. To be in communication with the leader of the Support Group and arrange occasional joint gatherings of Team and Group.

Getting Started

To ensure that this ministry is seen as the ministry of the whole congregation/parish, a formal Covenanting Service should be held. At this service, the persons involved should be named, prayed for, and commissioned for this particular ministry within the body of Christ.

When a Healing Team is ready to begin their ministry, the Worship Committee might be involved in deciding whether the initial healing service would best be informal or formal, with communion or without, with a printed bulletin or without, with an offering or without. The congregation/parish should have as much understanding and ownership of the ministry as possible. A Mission and Outreach Committee could also be involved at this stage, or later, to acquaint the community of the opportunity to receive healing prayer.

The healing/prayer team or Worship Committee, working with the Minister, could plan the first service. This could be well publicized in the church.

Those who attend should be invited to give feedback regarding the experience. On the basis of this feedback, and the participants' reflection on their own experience, further services could be planned at regular or irregular intervals. Continually evaluate these services. It is important to keep in touch with how the ministry is being perceived, and to give ongoing encouragement to the congregation/parish in general to attend and support the ministry.

Preparing for the Service

Sacred space is any space where the presence of the Holy is honored. But it is more than just "any space." Where healing is the desire and intention, the environment should be conducive to awareness of the presence of God who heals. Careful preparation of the space for worshipping and healing will express caring to people as they arrive, and prepare them to receive healing.

This means allowing ample time to set up the area. Avoid noise or hurrying around after people begin to arrive. Having chairs in place, table prepared, symbols (such as a Christ candle, cross, sculpture, Bible) set out, suitable lighting, flowers, comfortable temperature – all these assist in creating an atmosphere that is meditative, attractive, and welcoming. It instills a subtle message of confidence. It is also important that the greeters or ushers at the door be quietly warm and friendly, assuring, and able to respond to any initial questions a visitor might have.

Settings can vary: a living room in a home, a bedroom, a circle of chairs in a church school classroom or at the front of the sanctuary, a sitting room in a nursing home, a hospital room, the chapel of a jail, etc. Wherever we are moved by compassion and the Spirit to pray with heart and hands for healing is an appropriate setting. Jesus exercised his ministry of deliverance and healing anywhere and everywhere. And he still does.

Preparing the Healing Stations

Stations should be set up in the sanctuary – the places where members of the team will anoint, lay on hands, and pray. Usually, one station is prepared for each 10–12 persons expected to attend.

Each station will need a plate and cup for the communion elements if these are being used, and a container of oil. These will be brought from the Communion Table at the appropriate time in the service. Each station will need a small table for these. A box of tissues should also be placed within easy reach. A chair facing the chancel, or a kneeler at each station, will allow those who come to sit, kneel, or stand.

Stations should be set up far enough apart from each other and from those attending the service to ensure privacy. Ushers can keep those waiting for prayer at a respectful distance from the prayer station, to honor confidentiality.

Before the Service

Half an hour before the service begins, the healing/prayer team should gather with the worship leader to review procedures and to pray. As many members of the team as possible should join in prayer even though some may not actually lay on hands that particular day. At this time, any members who do not feel ready to act that day should have the option to say so.

Spend as little time on the mechanics of the service as possible, but be sure of clarity concerning:

1. Who will work as partners, and where their station is located.
2. If there is communion, which partner will serve bread and which wine or grape juice, and what words will be spoken as the elements are distributed. The worship leader or celebrant will assist with this.
3. Who will take the lead in anointing, and who in prayer time.
4. Who will be available near healing stations to care for any person needing special attention.

Preparing for Anointing

Prayer teams will have learned about the biblical and historical use of anointing in their preparatory study. But there are also practical aspects.

For example, the preparation of the oil. We recommend using pure olive oil. If you want a fragrant oil, do not add more than a drop of fragrance. Flower or other essences are very strong. Because some persons are allergic to perfumes, it is probably best not to use any fragrance. Members of the prayer team should personally refrain from using perfumes of any kind for the same reason.

Wayne and I once attended a healing service where pure, concentrated essence of rose was used as the oil for anointing. It was liberally applied. It ran down my forehead into my eye, which burned. Wayne said he "smelled like a rose for days!" That may have been an exaggeration, but in truth, the church and everyone in it reeked! So be cautious about the oil used. Even with olive oil, make certain that it does not become rancid, but is always fresh.

Any small, open container can be used for the oil. A small clay pot or a glass candle holder works well. The finger or thumb should merely touch the oil in the container and then be lightly wiped on the edge, so there is no possibility of the oil running down the person's face.

The sign of the cross is made on the person's forehead, with words such as the following:

- "I anoint you in the name of the Father, Son and Holy Spirit."
- "I anoint you in the name of God the Creator, Jesus the Healer, and the Holy Spirit."
- or simply "I anoint you in the name of God."

The words should be spoken reverently, the action unhurried.

If bread is served by the same person as the one doing the anointing, it is best to anoint with the second finger so that bread can be served with the thumb and first finger.

Laying on of Hands

Again, the healing team should have studied the history of this practice in Christianity, and understand its holy significance.

One or more members may lay on hands. Those trained in Healing Touch or Therapeutic Touch will understand that it is not necessary to actually touch physically, but still may choose to do so.

Although normally one would ask permission to touch, during a service people are specifically invited to come forward for the laying on of hands, so they will expect to be physically touched. Even so, one must be led by the Spirit in discerning whether hands on or off the body would be most helpful in each situation. For example, if a person requests prayer related to physical abuse, it would be probably best to pray with hands off. If a person is grieving the loss of a loved one, a light and loving touch on head, shoulders, or hand could add comfort to the words of prayer.

Where to place the hands reflects one's training and experience, but beginners should not feel anxiety about this. If one intends love, God's healing energy will flow from wherever the hands are, and it will flow where it is needed. One brings the hands to the head, shoulders, or upper back, or just holds the person's hands – whatever seems most natural.

Laying on of hands works best when working in partners. One partner will take the lead in offering prayer; either or both may lay on hands. The one not leading in praying should stand sideways and partially toward the recipient's back.

This partner should also watch for the well-being of the prayer recipient, particularly if the recipient is standing. Sometimes recipients feel faint, or move into an altered state of consciousness, sometimes called "being slain in the Spirit." If either of these happens, the watching partner must move quickly to catch the recipient, ease him/her to the floor without fuss, and arrange clothing as necessary.

For this reason, ample space must be allowed between the prayer station and the front pew. The person being prayed for may slump down, or fall forward or backward. Since the body is limp, the person will not normally be hurt in falling. But the person's head should not be allowed to hit the front pew! A person deeply resting in the Spirit may remain on the floor for some time, so a light cover may be needed for comfort as well as for decency. It is good to have a light cover folded, within easy reach.

In such a situation, the partners should proceed as usual to pray for others who come to their station. Meanwhile another prayer team member comes forward to sit nearby, to be prayerfully watchful, and to assist the resting person to arise when the time comes. It is important that the person rising should not experience any embarrassment, or be asked questions, but be quietly and lovingly attended to. At the end of the service, the prayer team member should be available if the person desires explanation or conversation.

Having a person "slain in the Spirit" may never happen in a service. But just in case, prayer team members must be prepared, and be calm throughout, remembering that since God is in charge, all is well.

Prayer for Healing In a Corporate Setting

Not all the words spoken in a prayer/healing service come from the prayer team members. Within the normal liturgy, we make our corporate approach and our communal confession. Often there is a period of silence for private confession.

The task of the prayer team is intercession. The person coming forward may wish to offer prayer aloud for himself/herself or for another. In this case the team partners may or may not add anything further. It is not necessary to repeat what has already been spoken.

Praying for healing for another is a sacred privilege. But remember always that the person praying does not do the healing, God does. However, words can "prepare the way for the Lord." They assist in centering. They bring the one being prayed for and the healing team into spiritual and mental resonance.

The choice of words of prayer in the healing service will depend on the situation. But whatever that might be, the personal preparation is the same. The essential preparation is the healer's own prayer life and daily close walk with God. As we learn to be comfortable talking to God and listening to God, as we practice some form of meditation, and as we learn to live attuned to God's presence, we grow in our personal relationship and we come to the ministry of healing out of that intimate relationship. This enables sensitivity both to the person coming for healing and to God who, through the Spirit, gives the words to speak. Having done this preparation, the healer's task is then simply to be quietly centered and open.

Those who come forward for prayer and healing may be invited to give their name. Some prefer to use the name in the praying, feeling it makes the prayer more personal. The person may also be invited to make a prayer request with such words as, "Do you wish to name a prayer concern?" or, more directly, "What is your prayer request?" Some may prefer, "What do you want Jesus to do for you?"

In making such a request, we follow the example set by Jesus himself:

> *There were two blind men sitting by the roadside. When they*
> *heard that Jesus was passing by, they shouted, "Lord, have mercy*
> *on us, Son of David!" The crowd sternly ordered them to be quiet;*
> *but they shouted even more loudly, "Have mercy on us, Lord, Son*
> *of David!" Jesus stood still and called them, saying, "What do you*
> *want me to do for you?" They said to him, "Lord, let our eyes be*
> *opened." Moved with compassion, Jesus touched their eyes.*
> (Matthew 20:30-34a)

The gospels tell us that Jesus often looked at a person and knew the need without a word having been spoken to him. So he did not ask for his own information, but that in answering the question the receivers might be fully open to receiving. It often helps the person coming for prayer to make a clear verbalized petition, and so to open that particular area to the healing action of the Spirit. The person offering prayer must listen very carefully to any words given, making no comment except, perhaps, asking for clarification. It's also important to attend to nonverbal messages, all the while remaining tuned to the Spirit.

In that scripture passage above, Jesus was moved with compassion. All our healing work must come from the same compassionate intention as Jesus'. A loving tone of voice is important in asking any question, so that the person coming feels no pressure. But sometimes the depth of feeling in the one who comes makes it too difficult to speak, or the issue may be too private or too sensitive to be shared in that moment. Public ministry is different than private ministry.

The Spirit may grant unexpected knowledge, by word or picture, but the spoken prayer may not reveal whatever the healer is given intuitively. With the gift of knowledge must also comes the gift of wisdom.

If no specific prayer is requested, and no particular intuition given, the healer prays generally for the healing and balance of the whole person. When many persons are present in a public healing service, it helps to give some forethought to the words used. This should be discussed during training with the prayer/healing team. Although prayer at all times must be guided by the Spirit, those laying on hands need to be clear about the essence of the prayer to be spoken. Prayers could follow patterns such as these:

- *God of Compassion, in your love, and by the power of the Spirit, restore balance in spirit, mind, body, emotions and relationships for this one of yours. And bless* (name, if known) *with your peace, in the name of Jesus Christ.*
- *Loving God, let your healing Light shine upon* (name, if known) *bringing wholeness in every area of being in the name of Christ the Healer.*
- *Lord Jesus Christ, lay your hand of healing upon* (name, if known) *that (s)he may live in wholeness, peace, and joy to the honor of your holy name.*
- *Life-giving God, let the love which flows from your heart to* (name, if known), *this beloved child of yours, bring new life, health and peace.*
- *Loving God, Giver of all good gifts, let your healing flow in the life of this dearly loved daughter/son of yours, and to you be all praise and glory.*

When offering a spontaneous prayer, a pattern can help:
1. Name God and offer a phrase of faith affirming who God is and what God is able and willing to do.
2. Offer a word of thanksgiving for the revelation of God's love in Jesus the Christ, and for God's love for the person being prayed for.
3. Make the petition.
4. Conclude with words of praise, giving the glory to God.

In general, pray positive, affirming, faith-filled prayer in words that are natural, sincere and loving, and leave the rest to God. In a public service, the prayers cannot be long. If a rote or formula prayer is used, its words, like any other prayer, must arise from a loving heart to be effective. The love, not the words, makes the difference.

When working with a partner, the two may simply take turns praying. Or they may sense by the Spirit's leading who should pray for a certain person. If a specific need is named and one partner has had more personal experience in that area, that person should take the lead in praying. Partners work best when they know each other well and can read each other's unspoken signals. The person not offering spoken prayer prays silently, supporting in silence the prayer being offered by the partner, and listening to the Spirit as well. The partner praying aloud should pause briefly before saying "Amen" to allow opportunity for the other to pray aloud – perhaps some intuition has come to the listening partner that is important to add. But the supporting partner never prays simply to be heard, or to repeat what has already been said!

Making the Best Use of Music

Music can assist in healing ministry, but music can be healing in itself. Music can be spiritually elevating. In addition, certain tones or frequencies may vibrate at a level affecting one or more of the chakras. They may also influence emotions, and affect the chemical secretions of the body.

When a person comes in, meditative music can aid in relaxing and quieting. Instrumental music without pronounced or startling changes in range, volume, or tone is best for centering and deep meditation. Background music, if used, should be quiet and instrumental, whether it comes from a musician, tape or CD. It is important to close with a hymn and/or prayer of thanksgiving, acknowledging with gratitude the Giver of all good gifts, including the healing received.

In worship, singing draws the community together and brings to remembrance God's love, power, and the Good News of the gospel. Chant is often useful for this purpose. Listening to hymns or choruses can be inspirational and affirming of faith. This heightens awareness of God's presence and goodness, and builds confidence in what God is able to do. A quiet Taizé-style chorus can also be a form of meditative prayer in preparation for receiving or ministering healing.

Some like to have choruses or hymns sung during the ministry time, because they cover the sound of the praying and so increase privacy. Ideally, however, every member of the group or congregation/parish should also be praying for each person as they are being ministered to by the prayer team. They can do this better without trying to sing at the same time.

Appendix E includes a list of suggested choruses and hymns.

Preaching

Preaching about healing is important, not only in healing services but from time to time in the regular church services. We need to hear the gospel word of love and forgiveness for sin; we need to hear that God does answer prayer! We need to revisit the healing stories of the Bible, to admit our own and society's need, and to hear the call to participate in Jesus' ongoing ministry. We need to be reminded of the difference between healing and curing, and of current prayer research that enhances faith. And we need to reflect with thanksgiving on our own experiences of God's faithfulness.

A homily and/or a word of witness should also be given in informal gatherings for healing prayer, because the Word proclaimed links the action of what we do to the action of Christ.

After the Service

Unless moved by the Spirit to continue to hold a person in our ongoing personal prayers, we simply release each one into the love and care of God as each leaves the healing chair, kneeler, or line. God nudged the person to attend the healing service. God encouraged the person to come forward. God is the healer in whose heart that person is continuously carried. Unless otherwise instructed, God expects us to let go!

After Praying

Here is an important principle. Believing that God has done the healing work appropriate, we do not return in thought or conversation to the condition as it was before prayer. If there is a refreshment time following a healing service, for example, we do not attempt to discuss further the reason or condition that brought someone to the service. We do not revisit what has already been committed to God in prayer.

However, if some do wish to talk further, we listen carefully. We may discern that they need further support. Lay people sharing in a healing ministry are not counselors, and should not undertake that role. If anything further appears to be called for, the person should be assisted to seek the counsel of a pastor or other trained individual.

From a practical perspective, prayer teams are likely not covered by insurance as are professional counselors, and so must be wary of giving anything sounding like formal counsel.

Incorporating Healing into Regular Worship

Most mainline churches entering into a healing ministry opt for a separate time of service from the regular Sunday morning hour. However, some congregations/parishes incorporate anointing and laying on of hands into the regular service, usually with communion. Persons come forward to receive the elements, and if they desire anointing, they move into a separate line to receive this ministry.

Other congregations or parishes have healing/prayer team members available at stations immediately following the regular worship service. Persons desiring prayer for healing wait in nearby pews and come as a station is available. In our experience, this method seems to encourage more in-depth prayer; usually more time is available than when healing is incorporated into the service itself.

Liturgy may be formal or informal, with communion or without. Sometimes prayers for healing can occur before the receiving of the elements, sometimes after. Holy Communion, when it is a part of the service, can be an act of celebration of what has taken place, or can open the spirit to God.

To introduce mainline worshippers to such services, it helps to maintain a liturgy that corresponds with what these people find familiar. Thus, they are not distracted by anxiety about what may be expected. Thom Davies, minister of Trinity United Church in Lively, Ontario, has incorporated healing prayer into the regular communion services of that congregation/parish. See Appendix F. Other healing service resources appear in Appendix D.

Broadening the Ministry

In-depth healing may not happen most appropriately in the public setting. In some churches, healing team partners meet by appointment for personal prayer ministry. There are also churches where bioenergy treatments are offered after church services, and churches where Healing Touch, Therapeutic Touch or Reiki treatments are offered mid-week and in homes, hospital and nursing home as requested.

If the ministry broadens to include bioenergy treatments given in the church, or if the congregation/parish sponsors a Parish Nurse program, the appropriate congregational body also needs to bring these under its oversight.

Some churches with healing ministries have follow-up opportunities during the week, following their Sunday healing service. At that time, persons come by appointment to meet with healing team members for private, in-depth prayer and conversation. It needs to be clear that this prayer ministry is not pastoral counseling or spiritual direction.

Other Groups

Some needs may arise which could be effectively met by a person attending some other kind of group for support. Support groups abound in the community outside the church, and many are initiated, led, or attended by church members. These are important groups and bring much healing into people's lives. However, there may still be a need for support groups – such as for grief, cancer, eating disorders, or parenting problems – where the church can add a spiritual dimension and perspective in an overt and intentional way. This can be missing in secular groups, and is important for healing of the whole person.

Parish Nursing Programs

It has long been known that there is a link between faith and health. To promote this understanding is part of the pastoral, educational, and mission mandate of the church. A number of churches now are instituting Parish Nurse programs. The parish nurse is concerned not just with the sick, but works within a congregation/parish and the surrounding community to assist the church in reclaiming its health ministry.

The parish nurse is a Registered Nurse on staff in a local congregation/parish. He or she works closely with the ministry team and the congregation/parish to promote health and wellness for the members, and for the community.

The parish nurse may provide Christian education on preventative health and well-being, for all ages. He or she may give pastoral care for people with specific health needs and for their families, and may act as liaison with healing agencies and community-based services. The parish nurse is a listener and advocate, assisting persons in dealing with life attitudes, stresses, losses, and griefs that, if unattended, can seriously affect wellness.

He or she could also relate to a prayer chain or prayer group, making intercessors aware of prayer needs and concerns in a congregation/parish and community. Perhaps a parish nurse might choose to be part of a healing/prayer team or to share in services of prayer for healing.

Parish nursing as a ministry is growing in Canada and the United States. It is proving its value alongside other professional leadership in the church.

Although all healing comes from God,
it is often mediated through a healer.
*Therefore, as **Rochelle Graham** explains,*
it is essential for the healer to provide the necessary self-care.
Healers too often think of themselves as givers, not as receivers.

12

Looking After Yourself

When there is so much need in the world, so much to do and so many asking for help, is it selfish even to contemplate self-care? Many people think of self-care as selfish-care. Instead, they care for others at their own expense. An old acronym promoted at Christian youth groups said, "JOY – Jesus first, others second, yourself last of all."

Jesus commanded us to "Love your neighbor as yourself." That calls for an equality of caring. Few of us manage that equality. Those with a Christian orientation are likely to love others and penalize themselves; those with a secular outlook may do the opposite.

In my workshops, when I teach the people to do healing work on themselves, I will often tell them, "Do this as though you are working on the most beloved person in your life." Many people respond to this with tears. It feels so wonderful to experience the love that they offer to others for themselves. Others respond with feelings of guilt: "How can I love myself? Is it self-centered to love myself?"

If we were truly to love our neighbors the way we love ourselves, it might be a world without much love.

Modeled on Our Heart

Our physical heart teaches us about self-care. It works nonstop as long as we are alive to keep us healthy and to take care of the whole body. It unites the many parts into one collective entity working in harmony. When the heart receives the blood from the lungs, it also receives the blood that the heart itself requires to be nourished and healthy, before it sends that blood out to the whole community. So in essence, with every beat, the heart receives first.

We can learn a lot from this wonderful organ. If we could only take time to make sure we are similarly nourished on all levels of our being before we care for others, we would have significantly more energy to care for others.

A good way to look at our own energy levels is to think of them as a bank account. You can't run on permanent overdraft. Every time you make a withdrawal, you need also to put in a deposit. Ideally, you would make the deposit before your withdrawal – most of us want to be sure the money is in the bank before we write a cheque! This means that you need to take stock of what kinds of things restore your energy – what builds you up and what depletes you. When you become conscious of this system of withdrawals and deposits of energy, you can then begin to live with balance.

My own discovery about self-care was a tough lesson to learn. I, my first husband, and our young son had just moved to a new community. Six weeks later, I gave birth by Caesarian section to a baby girl. Shortly after, visitors started arriving. I thought I had to be a gracious hostess, so I insisted on baking, cooking good meals, and ensuring our guests were well cared for. We had over 40 visitors during the next few months. Between caring for the new baby, my family and all the company, there was little time to care for myself.

That fall, the world was gravely concerned over the nuclear arms race. I felt that I needed to do something. I wanted to do everything possible to ensure that this world was a good place, a safe place, for my children to inherit. Through my church, I became very involved in "saving the world."

Within three years, my body was giving out. I was suffering from utter exhaustion, a kind of "battle fatigue." There were many factors involved in the breakup of that marriage, but I can say now that if I had known how to care for myself, and had believed it was important, the marriage might still have had a chance. But I was emotionally, physically, mentally, and spiritually bankrupt.

Strangely, in that bone-weary state, I began to hear the voice of God speaking more clearly to me. It said that through healing myself I would help in healing the world. What God needed most was not a worn-out shipwreck of a person, but a healthy, vital vessel. And so self-care became a priority.

This was not an easy transition for me. I had too many years of caring for others first, even to know how to care for myself. Learning how to ask for what

I needed was an enormous challenge. I found it easier to heal the world outside than to look at the world inside and own my internal pain.

The years following were painful and yet profoundly rewarding. Here is an excerpt from my journal, several years into my healing journey:

Gently I grow and blossom
as a rose unfolds its petals to show
the world its beauty.
I too am learning to slowly open
and share my inner gifts with the world.
I pray that I may continue to unfold
and allow my inner self to shine through.
May I love the world with all my heart
and may the love of God flow through me.
The candle within is shining brighter –
and I feel the warmth and light radiating outwards
to light the dark.

I know now that it is the deep emotional and spiritual healing I have done that allows me to journey with others as they face their inner wounds. I know now that when I care for myself, I am able to be a strong vessel for God, and I am able to travel as much as I do in teaching the Ministry of Healing. I still get tired. I still get depressed sometimes. But I know that I am able to help more people when I look after myself first!

Caring for the self means taking the time to know how you are doing on a physical, emotional, mental and spiritual level. It means knowing what you need and asking for it. It means recognizing that you are creating and maintaining a temple for God through your own being. It means diligently caring for your own body as a sacred space.

When you take time to pay attention to your physical body, you are honoring what the Bible calls the "clay vessel." The body has certain requirements to keep it healthy and filled with vital energy.

Rest

One of the first requirements for a healthy body is adequate rest. Every year when we begin daylight saving time, there are about 10 percent more motor vehicle accidents on the following morning than usual. Professor Stanley Coren attributes this increase to chronic lack of sleep, aggravated by the loss of one additional hour when we change our clocks. In contrast, when we regain the hour in the fall, the accident rate drops. As a society, we live on the edge of sleep deprivation.

Most people who come to see me are not aware of how tired their bodies are. They have been living at such a fast pace for so long that they don't know how to recognize the subtle messages of fatigue. The body almost needs to scream in exhaustion before we listen. When we are always running on "will power," we often don't feel our bodies at all.

Even ten minutes of horizontal time during the day will give our physical bodies an opportunity to rest, relax and recover. Wayne swears by "power naps" – ten minutes set on his watch so as not to be concerned about time, arms overhead to open up breathing, and feet elevated if possible. He says he can be asleep in ten seconds.

Exercise

Exercise and body movement are considered so essential to body healing that even in the Intensive Care Units of hospitals, patients are mobilized as soon as possible, sometimes while still attached to a breathing machine. Anyone who has had major surgery will remember someone coming to get them up for a walk; the effort to resist the pull of gravity is essential to minimize postoperative complications. The old saying, "use it or lose it," applies to our bodies.

Regular exercise oxygenates tissues better, improves blood flow, decreases heart rates, strengthens the heart, and generally helps the body to function more efficiently. Endorphins released during exercise improve the sense of well-being. This is also known as the "runners' high." In his book *Staying Healthy with the Seasons*, Dr. Elson M. Haas urges us to change exercise activities with the seasons. In very cold climates, when our metabolism is geared more for storage and preparation, activities like Yoga and T'ai Chi may be better. In spring, when a burst of vitality accompanies the increase in sunlight, our bodies will have energy for more vigorous activities.

Exercise doesn't need to be another chore, another "should" that we add to our list. The word recreation means re-create; it restores who we are. When we allow movement to take the form of play, we allow our beings to be re-created into wholeness. I have two favorite questions for my clients: " What kind of activities do you love?" And, "How often do you do them?" Most people's faces light up when they describe their favorite activities, and yet they rarely find the time to do them.

What is play to you? And how frequently do you play?

Many religious cultures use body movements as a form of prayer. In her book *Embodied Prayer*, Celeste Snowber Schroeder describes dancing as being a natural outpouring of spiritual joy. Celeste talks of the early Church as having dance and movement as part of worship. She quotes Augustine (354–430 CE) on dance as "bringing one's bodily members in accord with the love of God."

When we allow the divine within to move us, we move in harmony and in relationship with God. Even our breathing can become prayer when we welcome the divine in with each breath.

Diet

"We are what we eat," says a maxim. The food we eat nourishes the body as a sacred temple. Does that food honor or debase the temple?

What's the point of saying "grace" over food before eating? It could be just giving thanks. Or does the prayer honor and bless the food before it enters the temple?

When you begin to see the food you eat as food for the temple, you begin to consider more carefully the choices you make around food. There are so many choices to make about different diets, about what is healthy and what isn't, that at times choosing food can become yet another chore.

Here are two guidelines to consider:

How do you choose the food you eat? Is it simply by desire and habit? Or have you listened with wisdom to what your body really needs? James D'Adamo, the Toronto naturopath and nutrition researcher, offers a simple way to monitor the body's reaction to specific foods. He suggests fasting for three hours, taking your pulse, ingesting the particular food item, again taking the pulse, and charting this. It provides an indicator as to whether the body welcomes the food, or has to work to adjust to it.

Is the food prepared with love? Fast food and junk food are prepared as a commodity. Meals in the home may be offered in love – although, at times, they may not. How much time are you willing to spend in honoring the food and preparing it?

Eating is more than simply providing your nutritional needs. Like body movement, it too can become a form of prayer, of deeply honoring the source of all food and ensuring that the temple within is well cared for.

Fasting

Most of us consume foods and other substances through habit. We become, in effect, addicted. Fasting means examining those habits and abstaining from them until they no longer have power over us.

Choose habits that heal instead of harm. When a substance such as coffee, tea, or cigarettes has power over us, it limits our freedom. In essence, it holds part of our spirit hostage. When we find resistance to changing a habit, there is usually a large emotional component "below the surface," like the invisible bulk of an iceberg. By fasting or abstaining from that which has power over you, you allow the deeper issues behind the habit to surface for healing. The stronger the habit, the more it affects all levels of your being. Carolyn Myss, the author of *Anatomy of the Spirit,* tells of a person with AIDS. If she were to offer a cure for AIDS with one hand, and a cigarette with the other, she says, this individual would choose the cigarette. Smoking holds the person's spirit in a prison. In her book, she describes how important it is to open that prison and "call your spirit back."

Body Cleansing

Personal hygiene is another way of honoring and caring for the "clay vessel" that is the body. When you clean your body, do you lovingly wash all the parts as though they were the sacred temple?

Imagine if we were to wash our own feet as lovingly as the woman in the Bible washed Jesus' feet. Suppose you had the job of washing the sacred objects in your church, would you use care and reverence in the task? What about the special objects, the heirlooms and treasured souvenirs, in your home? Do the same with your body. When you step into the shower, allow the water to run over you, and offer prayers that this water be blessed as it cleanses this sacred vessel. Ask too that the water also cleanse your emotions, your thoughts, and your spirit.

Take the time to consider this as an act of healing, of restoration, of cleansing on all levels of your being. Your body knows and responds when it is lovingly cared for rather than washed simply for hygiene. Many people care for their cars, their lawns or their gardens better than they care for their bodies.

I recommend that after finishing giving a treatment, the healer wash his or her hands to release them from any residue of energy. In the same way, when Flora comes to the end of the day or the end of healing sessions, she often combines a prayer for cleansing with physical washing in a shower as a powerful restorative process. The flow of water through the aura assists in this restoration.

Mental and Emotional Self-care

Beyond the physical needs of the body, what about the way that emotions and thoughts affect us? Look at the metaphor of the bank account again. What stresses tend to empty your vitality or energy account? What fills your account so that "your cup overflows"?

Our bodies will signal us in many ways that we are stressed. Some people feel the "knot in their stomach," others notice the "pain in the neck." Unpleasant as these are, they can wonderfully warn us that our energy account is getting low.

A few years ago, I had a client diagnosed with multiple sclerosis. Through deep healing work over several years, he was able to become essentially symptom free. One leg still had minor sensory symptoms. These few remaining symptoms became his barometer indicating when pressure or stresses were getting too much. When the symptoms increased, the client knew to back off on his activities.

Many stresses are self-induced. We may have unrealistic expectations of ourselves. Many people have an abundance of "shoulds" in their life when what they need is an abundance of love and compassion for themselves. Often, we may still be playing old "tapes" in our heads or hearts – emotional recordings of people disapproving of our actions.

Other "old tapes" may be buried memories and unhealed wounds. Too often we "get on with life" rather than take the time to grieve, or to feel the pain and anger. But until we do, they still have power to bind us. It takes energy to keep struggling with all these old memories and emotions, and this can deplete the energy in our account. Pain, sadness, bitterness from years ago can color how we see life today. When the pain of an old memory interferes with life and generates stress in the present, it is valuable to seek professional help to assist in the healing process. Much of the healing work I do is helping people to release their old memories and stored emotions. Afterwards, they experience new life, new energy, and a new outlook on life.

You may have noticed that after spending time with some people, you feel restored. At other times, with other people, you feel extremely drained, as if someone had turned a vacuum on and sucked the vitality out of you. Keeping a healthy balanced energy account means being aware of those people who drain you and those who restore you.

If you need to give a lot in your work, and you feel very drained at the end of the day, how are you refilling your vitality account? Continued energy drain can be the cause of burnout in many of the caring professions. People give and give until they are bankrupt. Then they no longer have the energy to run their own bodies.

We need to listen to the symptoms of depleted energy sooner and take the steps to restore ourselves on all levels of our being. In her book *Prayer and our Bodies*, Flora Slosson Wuellner describes these symptoms as "angel messengers" that come to tell us that something is not okay. Before we take something to relieve the symptom, we need to listen to our bodies and the message the angel is bringing. Wuellner says, "This faithful, alert listening to our bodies is a holy and necessary part of our spirituality." Simply covering up the symptom doesn't cure the vitality deficit.

In listening, we honor our body's wisdom and honor ourselves.

Carrying Another's Burdens

Sometimes, in listening to our body, we realize that the pain we are carrying is not our own. When we have been present to someone who is in deep pain, it is easy to leave the situation "carrying their pain." Their story may have touched our story, and something we thought was over and done with in our past is once again very present to us. The challenge is then to sift through what pain belongs to you, and what belongs to the other person. Sometimes it is hard to know the difference, particularly if their story is similar to yours.

Being able to empathize with their situation may be valuable. But you can no more do their grieving or sorrowing for them than you can do their physical exercises. As helpers, we need to know ourselves well enough to know when to ask for help. We may simply need another person to debrief with, someone to help us sift through and discern what is ours and what is carried from the other person.

When we feel another person's pain, we are able to walk their journey with them and have deep compassion for what they are going through. But it does not serve either them or us to continue to carry that pain. When leaving a client or someone you have prayed with, it is essential to hand them over to God through prayer. We then release them, trusting that God will carry on with the healing.

Our editor Jim Taylor described their son Stephen's death. He and Joan, and their daughter Sharon, had gathered at Stephen's bedside for the three days of his final illness. During Stephen's last hours, just before he slipped into unconsciousness, Jim felt impelled to offer this prayer:

Dear God, this is Stephen.
We know that you know him already.
We know that you love him.
There's nothing more we can do for him.
So we turn him over to your hands, God.
Take good care of him, please.
For our sakes. Amen.

"It was painful," he says now. "We all cried. But I think it was helpful for all of us, and healing."

I have frequently worked with pastoral care workers or clergy who still carry years of other people's burdens in their hearts. Their hearts are stuffed full of other people's pain. Some have actually had physical symptoms, similar to those of various forms of heart disease, that were relieved only when these stories were released into God's hands.

We are not meant to carry the suffering of other human beings. God is.

Cast your burden on the Lord, and he will sustain you;
he will never permit the righteous to be moved.
(Psalm 55:22)

We are meant to be present, to listen, to care and love. And then we are to hand it all over to God and Christ, to transform the pain and suffering.

Come to me, all you that are weary and are carrying
heavy burdens, and I will give you rest.
(Matthew 11:28)

A helpful image might be to imagine the light and love of Christ or the Holy Spirit filling you and surrounding you as you listen and receive another's pain. As the other person releases this pain, it is absorbed and transformed by the light and love filling you and surrounding you. This way, it doesn't even have to go through you.

Renewal

Renewal in body, mind, and spirit is essential to anyone who works in a healing ministry. Each of us has to discover the ways in which we are nourished and restored on all levels of our being. This means doing a daily balance sheet of energy loss and energy gain.

I am restored by going up into the hills for a walk with my two dogs. There I can connect with the beauty, the peace, and the abundant energy of nature. I feel as though I open up, to release whatever I am carrying around with me, and to fill myself with the vital loving energy of Mother Earth.

For Wayne, renewal comes swiftly through deep listening to a variety of music. Flora is renewed by privacy and silence, nature, reading or cooking.

Nurturing the Spirit

Is it possible to look after yourself on a physical, emotional, and mental level, and still be bankrupt spiritually? In workshops, I ask that question. People can usually report how they are doing physically, emotionally, and mentally. But many people have no answers to the spiritual check-in. It is not because they don't have a spiritual self; it is mainly because they haven't put the energy or time into communicating with their spirit. They may not even know how!

The saints and mystics spent hours each day in prayer and meditation. Developing the connection to God was the essence of their lives. Today most of us rely on not much more than Sunday worship to feed the hunger of our spirit; we verge on being spiritually bankrupt. Most people spend more time being fed by the media than they do being fed by God.

Carolyn Myss differentiates between religion and spirituality. Religion, she says, is the community and belief system within which we practice our spirituality. For some this community and belief system may be supportive and nourishing; for others it may be toxic and stifling. For each person, each personality type, there will be methods of prayer, worship, and meditation that will fit best. Each person's spirituality forms a unique connection with the divine. Some people are met by God on a morning hike, some on the golf course, some when they stand in a stream with fly rod in hand. Our western culture is filled with people who have left their religion but are still hungry to feed their spirit. Others, wounded by the religion of their youth, have lost both their spirituality and their religion.

Many of the illnesses that I am called on to treat are actually crises of the spirit. These are people whose soul is calling out to be fed. Through the body, the soul is speaking. When the spirit is bankrupt, the body moves into crisis.

Our spiritual being calls out not only to be nourished, it calls out for wholeness and transformation. What are the ways that feed our spirit?

Spiritual Mentors

Reading about the different mystics and saints can help us to understand the many different approaches. We have a rich source of mentors and teachers through the stories of those who have gone before us. Wayne has found the biography and journal of John Wesley particularly helpful for him. My own mentors have included Hildegard of Bingen, the Sisters of Providence, and the Benedictine Order.

Through reading the experiences of others, we can gain perspective on our own spiritual journeys. Teresa of Avila's *Interior Castle* "jumped off the shelf" into Flora's hands 25 years ago; since then, Flora has read all her writings and regards her as a spiritual mentor. Studying the Rule of St. Benedict and learning Benedictine style (mantric) prayer, Flora discovered her most natural way of meditation. Benedict taught a rhythm of work and rest and prayer for every day that Flora considers essential.

Many persons find the spiritual journey of St. John of the Cross helpful, particularly in understanding the "dark night of the soul." And St. Ignatius of Loyola's teachings on meditating upon the life of Jesus as a prayer discipline have guided many into personal encounter with the living Christ.

Meditation and personal forms of prayer are ways either to begin or to support an ongoing spiritual journey. The styles of prayer and meditation we are drawn to pursue, reflect our personality type and stage of spiritual development.

When embarking on a spiritual journey, one of the most helpful guides is a spiritual director. This person can assist in the development of spiritual practices. In general, a spiritual director, guide, or companion is one trained to assist another become aware of, attentive to, and responsive to the movement and calling of God in the other's life.

A Sabbath for Rest and Renewal

The original concept of Sabbath was that one-seventh of our time was spent in resting and making space to connect with the divine. When Sunday worship becomes the only time that people spend in prayer, that time is cut down to one hour a week.

Our spirit requires much more time than one hour a week to be fed. Self-care for the spirit means to look at all the activities of a week, and determine which ones nourish the spirit, which ones deplete it, and which ones are toxic. Even washing the dishes can be prayerful when approached with that in mind. Brother Lawrence, in *The Practice of the Presence of God,* refers to the benefit of simple repetitive activity. This is a central concept of the Benedictines, who have functioned as a religious community for 1500 years. Every act in the day is a form of prayer to God, and work is a means to strengthen the soul. I found this quote from Teilhard de Chardin in Esther de Waal's book, *Seeking God: The Way of St. Benedict*:

> *God, in all that is most living and incarnate…is not far away*
> *from us…from the world we see, touch, hear, smell, and taste*
> *about us. Rather [God] awaits us every instant in our action, in*
> *the work of the moment…at the tip of my pen, my brush, my*
> *needle – of my heart and my thought.*

Prayer is whatever we do to connect with the divine. Appendix C identifies different styles and approaches to prayer. It is important that each person find the style that works best.

Meditation

The very word "meditation" still makes some Christians nervous. Not that long ago, there was a great fear that meditation – as promoted by the Beatles and the Mahareshi Yogi – was a Hindu plot to subvert the Christian faith.

Yet most of us have always practiced meditation, though perhaps not by that name. Flora was always drawn to daydreaming, for example. As a child, she would find her mind off on "flights of fancy" when, according to her teacher, she should be "getting down to work," or according to her mother, "doing something useful." Then too, there was that Bible verse about people being *"vain in their imaginations"* (Romans 1:21 KJV).

We now understand that imagination is a gift from God. It can be used to express creativity and also to pray.

What makes a practice Christian? Can jogging, dancing, following one's breathing, listening to music, or repeating a sound or word be considered Christian meditation? There can be mental, emotional and physical benefits to these. And there can also be spiritual benefit. But whether they are "Christian" or not depends on the attitude of mind and heart, on inner motivation. The Christian may be helped by asking, "Do I intend to have my whole being increasingly reflect the wholeness that is God's will for me? Do I desire that Christ be more and more formed in me?" The Christian healer can prayerfully ask, "Does this meditative activity serve to center me such that I may be a strong, clean, and clear channel of the healing power of Jesus?"

Meditation is a form of prayer. It can open us to the awareness of the presence of God, the love of God, the healing of God in a way that goes beyond vocalized or mental prayer. It can put us in touch with the Physician within. It is valuable not only for the healer who desires continuing inner transformation, but is recommended to others for the same purpose. Meditation is like entering into an inner sanctuary, a secret place. Jesus told his disciples:

> *Whenever you pray, go into your room and shut the door and*
> *pray to your Father who is in secret; and your Father who sees in*
> *secret will reward you.* (Matthew 6:6)

But since it is the "inner room" of being, meditation may be practiced in the midst of a crowd or on a busy street. It only requires setting one's attention to noticing God in the midst. One can meditate while reading the newspaper, or listening to the daily news – if in the process one reflects upon the interplay of forces in God's world, God's attitude toward the world, and our part in God's work in it. One can meditate upon the mystery of the universe in the beauty of a wayside flower, of a great piece of art, of music.

"Praying the scripture," as described in Chapter 8, is a way of actively using the imagination in meditation. It has its Christian roots in the teaching of St. Ignatius of Loyola, founder of the Jesuit order. It is one of myriad ways of meditation.

The purpose is the same, whether using a wide lens or a close-up. The meditator seeks by some means to move beyond the surface of life with its whirl of thoughts and actions and to enter a deeper level of mindfulness, by keeping the attention anchored in the present moment. It requires letting go of "doing" and surrendering to "being." In so doing, one can meet oneself in a more real way. Material stored in the personal unconscious rises to the surface. Meditation can be a means of inner transformation, or of revealing the shadow side of our nature and enlightening the darkness within. If there is a wall around the heart, meditation can soften that wall. It can bring us into heart-to-heart connection with the God of love. There is a place of peace inside every one of us, that place where we are connected with the divine, and meditation can lead us there.

A meditator gently but intentionally narrows the focus of the lens, to bring the mind to rest in the heart, where one comes before God in love and allows oneself simply to be loved. One may simply follow one's breath to the heart center or take a single word, phrase (*mantra*), or object and fully focus on it.

This narrowing and holding of attention is a kind of centering prayer which can lead to a deep union of one's spirit with the Spirit of God. This is known as contemplation. It has its Christian roots in the teaching of St. Benedict, John Cassian in the 4th century, and John Main in this century. A fuller explanation of mantric meditation is given in Appendix C.

Initially, the meditative path one can follow most easily depends to a considerable degree upon one's personality preferences. Each person has a preferred orientation toward meditation that primarily employs reflection (activity of the mind), or feeling(activity of the heart); imaging (engaging the senses) or non-imaging (moving beyond the senses). The most helpful means of meditation may change as one progresses in the spiritual life, and one may find that in time one is drawn to the opposite of the initially preferred style. These things one must search out for oneself or with the help of a spiritual director.

To receive the benefit of meditation, though, one must practice it daily. Twenty minutes morning and evening is recommended, though there is still benefit in shorter periods. But more than 30 minutes is not recommended.

Each person must determine where and when is best for regular times of meditation. As with prayer, find time when you will least likely be disturbed. Take the telephone off the hook, or at least turn off the ringer. Your meditation time is worth it.

There are four sample guided meditations in Appendix C.

Journaling

Recently I reviewed the journals I have kept for the last ten years. As I read them, I realized these journals are the record of a profound healing journey. They hold the stories of my dreams, my visions, my pleas and lamentations, my conversations with God. At times the pages recorded my anger and rage. Other times they absorbed my tears as I wrote about the griefs in my life. There are pages of joy and celebration.

Some pages look like a little child got hold of them – because a child did. Those pages hold the stories of the wounded child within. There were times when the pages of the journal allowed me to process what was really going on; it let me vent in a safe manner; it let me clear my thoughts and emotions. Always, they provided me with an opportunity to understand myself better.

Most of all, in looking back over the volumes that I wrote, I can deeply honor the aspects of myself that called out for healing and wholeness. I can cherish the ups and downs of this spiritual journey called life.

When we embark on this path, the path of being an instrument in healing, it is essential for us to make a commitment to personal self-care and personal development. In keeping track of ourselves, we can monitor what our needs are. We can keep track of how we've changed.

In midlife, as Flora rereads the journals of a lifetime, she says,

> *I can see how God has been with me,*
> *how I have been held as I struggled and searched,*
> *questioned and doubted, hoped and dreamed, grieved and*
> *celebrated. I can see there has been meaning in it all.*
> *And I am helped to reflect on where I am now,*
> *and the changes I am experiencing,*
> *knowing there is meaning still.*

Journaling can be a very helpful tool to facilitate the process of knowing ourselves better. It is a way of charting the journey, of keeping a map of where we have been.

There are many different forms of journal writing. My own kept track mainly of my deepest thoughts, emotions, and archetypal energies. Other people keep dream journals, where they record their dreams and the teachings that come through them. Some keep prayer journals.

But remember that a journal is not a diary. A diary is a record of daily events; in a journal, one reflects on these events, noticing one's response to them, noticing what is stirred up inside by them.

Henri Nouwen says in his *Genesee Diary* (really a journal),

> *I have little to say about events, good and bad,*
> *creative or destructive, but much to say about*
> *the way I remember them – that is the way I start giving them*
> *form in the story of my life.*

A journal is a mirror in which we see ourselves and discover who and where we are.

If journal writing is new to you, here are some simple guidelines to help you begin.

- Find a quiet, private space where you will feel comfortable writing. Remember that journals are confidential unless you choose to share them.

- Don't worry about neatness or penmanship. Freedom to express what is inside is more important than how the page looks.
- Allow all aspects of yourself to be expressed on paper. Self-knowledge and self-healing means that we have to face all those parts, even those parts that may be jealous or bitter. Ignore old tapes that tell you, "If you can't say anything nice, don't say anything at all." Writing about those aspects of ourselves that we don't like allows us to bring them to the surface for healing. It also helps us to ensure that we aren't projecting those unwanted emotions onto others. When we find ourselves disliking someone, the journal grants a perfect opportunity to sift through what is being provoked and revealed in our inner selves. When we can see our inner wounds with compassion, it allows us to respond compassionately to others with the same wounds.

Support Groups for Healing Ministry

While many of the self-care activities in this chapter can be practiced alone, a support group can provide both nurture and continuing education. Whether it is a prayer group, a healing group, a meditation group, or a combination of these, a support group will encourage you to keep going.

By having others with whom to share experiences, you can learn from the ups and downs of developing new skills – theirs, and yours. A support group also offers opportunity for discernment. Here is a chance to say, " I experienced this while I was meditating. Have any of you ever had that happen?"

Personally, I have found support groups essential in developing the art and skill of hands-on healing. It provides a safe place to practice the skill and to get feedback from peers prior to offering any healing method to the wider community. An added benefit of a regular practice session is that you yourself also receive healing regularly.

It is important with support groups to stay focused on why you meet. If a group simply becomes a social gathering and the original intent becomes lost, people will begin to drift away. Here are some guidelines.

- Ensure that some standards determine how your group will function. How will the room be set up? What will the environment be like and who is responsible? How are decisions made? Who is leading – or is it shared leadership? How does each person give input? Will there be fees to cover costs?

- Define the group's purpose and task clearly. This way everyone knows why they are there and what to expect from the time together. Usually this includes specifying the length of time involved.
- Help to ensure all individuals have their needs met, and that each person is welcome. If certain needs are beyond the scope of the group, state that clearly. Unless it is a therapy group with trained leadership, a support group is not usually the place for therapy.

Continue Learning

Most professions recognize the importance of continuing education, keeping up with what is new. The same applies to healing ministry. Despite all the books available, healing work is similar to an apprenticeship. There is much to learn from someone who has walked this journey before you.

One of the most important ways to continue your learning is through a mentor. A mentor has the skills and knowledge you desire and is willing to journey with you, assisting you on the path. I have formally acted as a mentor for over 30 people and informally for many more. I make a commitment, usually for one to two years. We contact each other monthly through phone, fax, e-mail, or in person where possible. We discuss clients, personal growth issues, and techniques. They learn through receiving information handed down personally, and I learn from their learning. Much more is transferred than could ever be learned through books.

The goal of any mentor, of course, is to prepare those who have been mentored to mentor others. This way, learning is continually passed on, and more people are supported in developing as healers.

One of the tasks I give my "mentees" at the beginning of the formal process is a self-study. They reflect on their current level of knowledge, where they are in skill development, and how they are doing physically, emotionally, mentally and spiritually. From this, they set goals for the next year. These include personal healing as well as learning goals.

This is a useful task for anyone to do. I recommend it to you, whether or not you seek to be a healer in the Christian tradition. Each year, set aside time to consider your current mental, physical, emotional, and spiritual state. From that, determine the areas in which you would like to improve. Then find the books, the workshops, and the teachers who will meet those needs.

Despite all the evidence, all the experience, and all the history of healing,
we still don't know what actually happens.
Perhaps, suggests **Wayne Irwin**, *there will always be aspects*
of this ministry that we will never understand.
But that need not stop us from continuing to work with the mystery.

13

Always a Mystery

One of the first occasions when I laid hands on someone in a formal public healing service was during an evening gathering in Lowville United Church, in Burlington, Ontario. Persons from various prayer groups in churches in the area were gathered for mutual support. A young man stepped into the sanctuary. As he did so, an elder whispered to me, "That person coming in is emotionally disturbed; his mother has brought him tonight for healing prayer."

When the moment came for those desiring prayer – for themselves or for another – to come forward to receive the laying on of hands, the young man approached me, and knelt.

As I placed my hands near the young man's head, an inch or two above his hair, the palms of my hands felt as though I had placed them upon a mound of squirming worms. I had not touched the young man at all.

Nor did I touch him as I prayed. I spoke words of affirmation of the love and power and healing will of God, asking for the fullness of God's gracious blessing. And as I did, I noticed that the squirming under my hands began to ease. By the time I had concluded my prayer with thanksgiving, the buzzing sensation seemed completely calmed. The young man stood, smiled, and murmured, "Thank you."

At that time, I knew nothing of the theories concerning the "brain waves" of the planet – the so-called Schumann frequencies. I knew nothing of the "buzz" of out-of-phase vibrations between the electromagnetic energy fields of the person praying and the recipient. In fact, I knew next to nothing about the whole concept of the energy fields of the body. My only exposure to the "aura" had been in portraits of saints and others with haloes, in stained glass windows and classic paintings.

I did know of the ancient church tradition of prayer for healing. I had read the affirmation of the Book of James, in the Bible, that *"the prayer of faith will save the sick."* Out of that faith, and that faith alone, I was conducting this ministry. And it was enough. It is always enough to simply offer whatever you have to offer out of the strength of the faith, the love and the compassion that God has brought to life within you.

We Do Not Know All We Think We Know About Life

In the years since then, I have engaged in much study of the theology, the physics, and the metaphysics of prayer for healing. I have tried to understand what can be understood of the theories – spiritual and secular – that attempt to explain the mystery of our human experience. But every question answered tends to raise so many more new questions – some that we humans never knew enough to ask before. Whatever we learn about how things operate only pushes me to new levels of faith, and moves me to marvel all the more at the wonder of this life, this world, the worlds beyond, and at the mystery of how God has made us and everything that is. As the Psalmist expresses it, we are *"fearfully and wonderfully made"* (Psalm 139:14). As soon as we think we have everything sufficiently figured out, something else reminds us that we really do not know what it is we think we know.

Especially in these times when the scientific mindset dominates our culture, when television offers instant analyses of events, when we expect immediate explanation of all occurrences, human pride often deludes us into believing that humanity can now answer every question, that anything that can occur already has, and that there is truly "nothing new under the sun."

In Ecclesiastes 1:10, the writer known as "The Teacher" wrote,

> *Is there a thing of which it is said, "See, this is new"? It has already been in the ages before us.*

In this book, we affirm that same philosophy. We have limited vision and abject poverty of awareness of the infinite magnitude of the awesome mystery of loving reality, both human and divine.

Light is Still a Mystery

Everyone knows what "light" is. It's what the sun puts out. It's what you get, along with heat, when you start a fire.

In school, we learned the conventional theories about light, developed by Isaac Newton. Back in the 17th century, he established the scientific method – the combination of ideas, observation, and experiment on which modern science stands. Much of our culture today is rooted in the thought of this great man. Our understandings of how the world works, of how the human body works, even how the world economy works, are built largely on the notions of Isaac Newton. So we are very reluctant to entertain the thought that some of Newton's convictions have had their day.

Newton, however, was not above questioning the established wisdom of his own day. He dared to test some long-standing ideas, specifically those of Aristotle, the ancient Greek philosopher, who had declared many centuries before that white light was light in its pure unadulterated form, and that color was a defilement of that light.

Newton questioned those assumptions about light. White light, he discovered, was not pure light at all, but rather a mixture of the many colors of the rainbow. Newton's conclusion upset an understanding of reality that had endured since before the days of Jesus. Furthermore, Newton had accomplished his coup by a rigorous new experimental method of testing that he had designed himself, the findings of which appeared to be unassailable.

Newton, in fact, established the very first truly scientific model of reality. He showed that the universe obeys certain laws of behavior; everything observes a rule of "effect following cause." In other words, according to Newton's theories, anything that happens can ultimately be predicted; the universe behaves like the unwinding of a giant clock.

In the centuries since Newton, most of our common beliefs about reality have been based upon these concepts. But by the beginning of the 19th century, his opinions of light were also being challenged. Newton had postulated that light was made up of corpuscles or particles. Others, using Newton's own experimental methods, now suggested that light might not be made up of particles; they showed it to behave as a wave form.

New Notions of Space and Time

Michael Faraday, considered the greatest experimental scientist of the 19th century, demonstrated that light moves like waves – sometimes. Faraday also developed the related concept of "fields of energy," the concept that has become a model for today's understanding of how various seemingly separated objects in the physical universe are actually connected to each other.

A contemporary of Faraday, James Clerk Maxwell, developed another theory, that light is a form of electromagnetic radiation. Earlier philosophers had thought light to be an emanation from the eyes. Light did not come *to* the eyes; it reached out *from* the eyes into the world around, much like a blind person's white cane "feeling" the environment.

And then Max Planck, a German physicist, pursued the mystery of light radiating from hot objects. He found that wave theory alone could not explain this phenomenon. He could explain it only by supposing that light was emitted in "packets of energy" of a definite size. He chose to call the packets *quanta*. His announcement launched a revolution in science that would come to be known as "quantum physics."

About this time, Albert Einstein graduated from the Technology Institute in Zurich. Einstein asked himself: "Suppose one took a ride on one of these packets of energy, on one of these *quanta*. How would the universe look to a person riding on a quantum, and would that person experience the flow of time?"

He suggested that the person riding on the quantum would seem to be still while all other objects rushed by at the speed of light. It would be the same effect as if the distance between all objects being approached had been reduced to zero. For the person on the quantum, either time would seem to not exist, or distance would have no meaning. Time and distance were intimately related.

The Implications for Healing

This idea of Einstein's, now a century old, is of great interest for our present consideration of the mystery of the effect of prayer for healing at a distance. The popular idea attributed to Einstein that nothing can ever travel faster than the speed of light is in fact incorrect. Einstein did not make such a statement. It was not part of his relativity theory. What he did say was that according to his calculations, it was impossible for anything to cross the speed-of-light "barrier." If something did exist that could travel faster than the speed of light, it would always have to remain traveling faster than the speed of light. It would also have to possess the characteristic of traveling backward in time.

As strange as this concept may seem, faster-than-light particles have been embraced as a possible explanation for other mysteries in theoretical physics. These imaginary entities have been dubbed "tachyons" – their name deriving from the Greek word meaning "swift." No one has ever seen or proven their existence, but the idea made the theory of moving backward in time a possibility, which, in turn, has come to relate directly to the work of Robert Jahn.

Jahn, with the Princeton Engineering Anomalies Research (PEAR) program, is presently demonstrating in the laboratory that loving intention, after the fact, can have a measurable effect on the behavior of inanimate objects with a random variable component, even when the intention takes place up to four days later. He is presently exploring the effect of the emotions of groups on the output of a piece of electronic instrument sitting in their midst.

The Mystery Continues to Deepen

Planck's *quanta* came to be known as "photons." But it took more than 20 years before the theory of how electrons and electromagnetic radiation interacted with each other would engage public interest. It fell to Richard Feynman, in the mid-20th century, to present this interaction in an understandable way. He described what he called "the strange theory of light and matter," or more technically, "quantum electrodynamics." Mathematically, he showed that time has no meaning for a photon. Also, with enough energy a photon can turn itself into what at first appears to be two particles: an electron with a negative charge and a positron with a positive charge. But this can equally be interpreted as the photon turning itself into only one particle, an electron that is sometimes moving forward and sometimes moving backward in time.

Quantum electrodynamics has turned out to be the most successful and seemingly most accurate scientific theory there has ever been. It explains everything in the physical world except gravity and the behavior of atomic nuclei, and it has been tested to an extraordinary degree of precision in experiments. Feynman and two others were awarded Nobel prizes for its development in 1965.

The theory has supported experiments in the 1990s showing how photons can behave as both particle and wave form at the same time. It has enabled further work to show that photons can appear out of what seems to be "nothing at all," or as Genesis (1:2) puts it, out of *"a formless void."* Physicists in New Zealand are now working on the illusion of distance, attempting to show experimentally that a single photon can exist in two different places in the same moment in time.

In spite of all of this, the mystery remains. Three centuries have passed since Newton first challenged the ideas of Aristotle, but although everyone believes they know what light is, even today, no one can technically answer the question, "What is light?"

The mystery persists. And with it persists the question of the nature of reality itself.

New Understandings of Reality

From the search for the nature of light has arisen a new question – how forces affect objects at a distance.

Newton realized that gravity acted at a distance. An apple high in a tree was attracted by the ground below, though the ground had no visible connection with the apple. To Newton it seemed so mysterious that he referred to gravity as an "occult force" – not in the popular sense that it was "evil," but in the true sense of the word, that its nature was hidden.

David Bohm, a brilliant physicist, philosopher, and explorer of consciousness, put forward a new explanation in this century. Bohm believed that science alone could not describe these connections between objects. In the 1970s, he was testing some of Einstein's presuppositions, and building on the work of Bell whose theorem, referred to in Chapter 10, had upset Einstein's conviction that subatomic entities exist independently of each other.

Bohm proposed that distant objects are actually related by their "consciousness" in a way that classical physics cannot explain. He used the term "nonlocality" to describe interactions that appear instantaneous, transcending space and time.

He added that one of the barriers to understanding this new insight concerning reality is our language. The way we speak is a traditional pattern with emphasis on nouns rather than verbs. This maintains the assumption that objects are separate from each other. Our whole language structure, he said, is founded on notions of location and separateness rather than of constant movement, connectedness, and flow. And yet life is an "unbroken, undivided process of flow," Bohm asserted.

The Broader Theory of Consciousness

Bohm was building on a concept of consciousness advanced by engineer and philosopher Itzhak Bentov and others. Bentov, in *Stalking the Wild Pendulum*, defined consciousness as the capacity of any system to respond to a stimulus. Even an atom, when it becomes "excited" by ultraviolet light, for example, could be considered to have a measure of consciousness – a primitive one, to be sure.

Bentov further theorized that the normally accepted human view that a rock, for example, does not have consciousness reflects our understanding, not necessarily reality. No one, he said, has ever proven that consciousness is actually limited to systems that have human or animal life. But humankind has decided to believe, arbitrarily, that consciousness belongs only to entities whose behavior resembles our own.

Bentov argued that consciousness – at least by his definition – is characteristic of all matter. Traditional biology has treated multicellular plants and animals as complex pieces of machinery. It has described them as "organisms." It has identified the physical components that apparently control their organization. But traditional biology has severely limited the response it is prepared to believe possible for each entity.

This stand has begun to be shaken. Bentov went so far as to suggest that awareness, on a scale that runs from "primitive" to "refined," is an attribute of every object, microscopic or otherwise. This phenomenon may explain the inclination of human beings to sense a harmonic response in such things as solitary trees and standing stones, for example, which were known in ancient times as "sacred places." The gratitude of an animal finding shelter under a mighty tree, or the relief felt by a bird resting on a standing stone, Bentov said, would linger and accumulate, enhancing the level of consciousness of that particular inanimate entity. Something special beyond the physical was going on. And a sensitive human being later approaching this place would feel the remnants of that "something special," and attribute some of it to the presence of a spirit.

David Bohm's ideas incorporated these understandings, addressed some of the old questions, and then raised new ones:

- Is our consciousness separate from that of others, or are we actually all of one mind?
- Is our human consciousness separate from that of other creatures, from that of other cellular structures, or are we all actually a part of the Mind of God?
- Is our awareness simply our own, or is it an aspect of the awareness of God? Is everything, including the past and the future, actually enfolded into the "now moment"?
- Do we, in fact, have access to every fragment of information within creation at every moment, in every place, wherever that might be? And if so, is it possible that all we really need to learn is how to log in to the universal database of intelligence?

Bohm found an analogy for his questions in the hologram – the form of photography in which the entire scene is contained in each tiny portion of the photographic plate. Any piece of a hologram picture actually contains all the information about the whole.

The Idolatry of Science

In recent years the dividing line between physics and metaphysics has become more and more indistinct. The old ideas about the true nature of reality have been foundering. The scientific method pioneered by Newton has been a life raft for those unwilling to face the prospect of continuing mystery. Traditional science itself has become an idol, a pagan god, a power to invoke whenever necessary to protect the status quo. True mystery is banished by this god, as though enigma and paradox and the unprovable must no longer be allowed to exist.

Many within the church have fallen under the spell of this spirit. Miracles are no longer expected. Even in the church, the Newtonian worldview – that cause and effect must always hold sway, that everything is rational and predictable – is held as dogma.

This view seems to be especially rigidly held when it concerns disease. Such persons argue that healing ministry should be simply left to conventional medicine. They are clinging to an outdated understanding that is now being challenged even by doctors themselves who have come to know the benefit of healing prayer.

Actually, true miracles do still happen. They happen not in contradiction to nature, but, as St. Augustine put it, "only in contradiction to that which is known to us in nature."

I recall a former parishioner who suffered an aneurysm of the brain. He was admitted to the hospital with what the doctors called a "zero chance of recovery." His family camped in the intensive care waiting room, praying for him at a distance, and sitting with him when they could, holding his hand, talking with him, encouraging him aloud, telling him of their love for him. They could visit physically with him for only five minutes every hour – the maximum time that hospital rules allowed. But they kept it up for a full two weeks, spelling each other off, until he finally awoke from his coma.

"Every time I see you, you are looking better," were my first words to him.

His first words to me, in response, were, "Too bad I can't say the same about you!"

He recovered. How come? Who knows? There was mystery. But there was surely healing, too, from the heart of his family.

We Do Not Know What We Do Not Know

We think we know what we know. We truly have no idea what we do not know. In our healing ministry within the church, we can be encouraged by realizing that as wonderful as traditional science is, it nevertheless has clay feet. Experimental methodology is not our god. The divine reality revealed in Jesus is able to do "new things." And new things happen all the time.

Science is certainly a valuable way of making some kind of sense out of what we observe. But it is not a god. It does not know all the answers. It does not have a handle on the whole truth.

In science, every theory only lasts until a better one comes along. Elmer Green, a co-founder of biological feedback research, puts it provocatively – a theory, he says, is "a set of blinders by means of which the left cortex focuses attention on what it wants to see." We cannot perceive all the information available to us without a "noise filter," a theory that puts the evidence into place. But for any particular theory, anything that does not get through the filter, that doesn't fit, is discarded. It is counted as just "noise."

And yet all such noise, when properly understood, is actually other information. It may not filter through the theory, but it still exists. So, says Green, "it is useful to remember that all theories will either change, or be abandoned, or be absorbed as special cases of more general theories."

No one has been able to develop the long-sought "theory of everything," and such a theory may never be possible. John Barrow, in *Theories of Everything*, points out that even the most comprehensive mathematical explanation cannot account for the differences in human experience. Mitchell Waldrop, in *Complexity*, raises some of the great questions that no theory has answered, and possibly that no theory will ever be able to answer.

- How did the primordial soup of amino acids and other simple molecules turn itself into the first living cell?
- Why did individual cells begin to form alliances?
- What can account for the development of such wonderfully intricate structures as the eye or the kidney?
- What, in fact, is life?
- And what is mind?
- What is thought, or purpose?
- Or what is feeling?
- And why after all these millennia is there actually something in existence, rather than nothing, since everything has the tendency to deteriorate and decay?

A Gross Oversimplification of Reality

All scientific doctrine is, in fact, a simplification of this mysterious complexity. It depends on approximations and unprovable assumptions as a base for all so-called "proven" theories. Gregory Bateson, the renowned anthropologist and philosopher, has aptly stated that prediction can never be absolutely valid; science can never therefore *prove* any generalization or even test a single statement in a way that arrives at a final truth. We can record the color of a million crows, each one black. We can issue a statement of theory that all crows are black. But it takes only one anomaly – the appearance of a single white or gray crow – to remind us that our theory is not absolute truth.

Everything we know is limited by a threshold. We can only see so far. We can only detect certain things. We can only measure for so long. Put the Hubble telescope into space, or put Sojourner, the robot laboratory, onto the surface of the planet Mars, and our threshold is extended. But, in truth, we cannot predict what will happen in the very next instant. Princess Diana dines out in Paris, and moments later she is dying inside a smashed Mercedes.

We also cannot foretell everything that will be discovered as we probe the next level of our knowledge. We can make educated guesses based on what we have observed in the past, but that is all that they are.

So when we pray for healing, the outcome can never be definitively known in advance. And one of our tasks within the healing ministry of the church is to guard against restricting that outcome, by refusing in our praying to focus our minds exclusively on what the world presently declares to be the limits of what is possible. Only God knows what is possible: *"with God all things are possible."*

Gordon Schwartz, a lay Jewish philosopher and dear friend of mine, puts it this way:

> We must never lose sight of the wonder of the mystery.
> Every religion has limited its people by attempting to put wraps
> around its teaching, and to presume to declare that it has within
> its dogma the answer to all questions.
> We are not here to know all the answers to all the questions.
> We are here to explore and to enjoy the mystery.

Whatever we know of God through our relationship with Jesus is, for us in the church, a sufficient revelation of the nature of God, not a complete one. We can never even manage to fully know ourselves, let alone fully know a family member or a friend. We gain sufficient knowledge of each one to be in relationship with them, to enjoy their presence in our lives, to feel blessed by them. But even another human being is too complex an entity for us to know in totality, let alone to know the paradoxical and unbounded infinitude of God. William Blake, in his poem *Auguries of Innocence,* penned these lines:

> *To see a World in a grain of sand,*
> *And a Heaven in a wild flower,*
> *Hold Infinity in the palm of your hand,*
> *And Eternity in an hour.*

Seeing with the Skin

Muse on the mystery of Rosa Kuleshova. Rosa, a young woman living in the Soviet Union in the early 1960s, could see with her skin. With her eyes completely covered, with credible witnesses present, in public, and in the company of representatives of the western media, she identified the main colors on the covers of two magazines by sensing them with her fingertips.

Before she did it, she asked someone to hold their hands over her eyes, even pressing on their hands herself with her free hand, stating, "If any light gets in, it distracts me."

Rosa identified the colors correctly, first by gently rubbing the surface of the magazines. She then repeated the demonstration with two other magazines, not touching them, but holding her hands six inches above them. And when a skeptical journalist placed his business card in front of her – something she could not have possibly ever seen before – she read everything on it, including the fine print, word for word, without a mistake, using not her fingertips, but her elbow!

Rosa's story was so compelling, it was accepted for publication, along with photographs, in *Life* magazine. Rosa's ability was given a name by the scientists who experimented with her, and subsequently with many others. They called it "dermo-optical perception." As might be expected, the concept was received with responses that ranged from scorn to enthusiasm.

Rosa insisted that her ability could be taught. It stretched belief, yet it was soon demonstrated. With six months of practice, others found they too could see with their hands.

The idea that we have only the five traditional senses – sight, hearing, taste, smell and touch – is another major oversimplification. The touch sensors involved in distinguishing hot from cold, for example, are different from those involved in distinguishing hard from soft. The taste buds that detect sweetness and bitterness are different from those involved in sensing saltiness. Yet they are all considered to be only one sense. We have no way of naming the way we sense anger in a room, trouble with a family member at a distance, or pleasure at the sight of a sunset. All these involve sensing in other ways.

The Human Body Can Control the Energies of Nature

The mystery of Rosa Kuleshova might ultimately have been dismissed as an anomaly, an aberration. Except that a decade earlier, a Russian psychologist named Alexei Leontyev, following in the tradition of Pavlov's famed work with dogs, had attempted to explore the human ability to be conditioned to react to a physical stimulation that could not be consciously sensed. The subject placed a finger on a key, and had to remove it the instant a green light was flashed upon his or her palm to avoid a shock. Leontyev found that the sensors in the palm of the hand could tell the difference between a flashed green light and a red one.

Does this astonish you? Then you may remember the astonishment of the disciples at Jesus' ability to walk on water, at his feeding of the 5,000, at his turning water into wine. And we in the church could remember Jesus' rebuke of his disciples, when he stilled the storm with a word: *"Why are you afraid? Have you still no faith?"* (Mark 4:40).

Elmer Green, the co-founder of biofeedback, declares that we have all been conditioned by our western culture, by the philosophies underpinning our education that mind and body are separate, and by the social leadership that believes that we know what we actually do not know. He states that we have succumbed to the temptation to believe the satanic lie that we are powerless to control or change whatever is happening in our bodies or in our lives, or in those of any others who are close to us. We have forgotten the primacy of the heart and mind connection.

Traditional psychology has taught us that our actions reflect only our genetic inheritance and our environmental conditioning. Traditional medicine has taught us that the doctor is the one who always knows what is best. And traditional medical treatment, at least in North America, has an extremely narrow view of illness, turning mostly to drug treatment, surgery, and radiation. As Green describes it, no one has officially informed us that our bodies tend to do what we tell them to. We have lost touch with the core of the mystery, that somehow everything in nature is connected to the heart and the mind.

Robert Jahn spent a decade with his Princeton Engineering Anomalies Research program exploring the interaction between human consciousness and the physical world. Just as Einstein revealed an association between energy and matter, so Jahn is now demonstrating a connection between thought and energy. His work, along with that of some others, is forcing science to take seriously the influence of the observer upon the observed.

That influence has been known and accepted in dealing with subatomic particles – but not with living beings.

Austrian physicist Erwin Schrödinger published a famous puzzle as far back as 1935, in which he played with this mystery of the influence of the observer upon what is observed. His puzzle was designed to suggest the absurdity of the concept, but instead, confirmed the theory. The puzzle was called "Schrödinger's Cat." It involved a thought experiment in which a cat in a room either lived or died depending on whether an observer could see an electron in a particular box. Because an electron was technically understood to be really only a cloud of the possibility of energetic forces, rather than an actual particle, being observed forced it to materialize.

The intent of the puzzle was to prove that the cat, like the electron, was neither alive nor dead, but only possibly one or the other, until the observation was made. The act of observing crystallized the reality.

Taking this understanding to its limit seemed ultimately to prove that the universe itself was neither physically real or not real until it was observed. It implied that creation itself could only exist if there were an outside "observer."

I believe that as we observe the condition of our own health, of our own wellness or illness, or even of the state of our own relationship with God, we similarly crystallize that condition. That is, we make substantial what otherwise might well remain suspended indefinitely. I knew an elderly man in one of my congregations who refused to see his doctor. He knew that the doctor, as observer, would give him a diagnosis. As long as his health condition could not be defined, his life could continue without having to address some named infirmity. Living with the mystery, for him, was better than having to face a known disorder.

The Beneficial Effect of Loving Ourselves

Jesus taught his disciples that they should love one another. Little could they imagine that the day would come when technology would measure the beneficial effect of such love upon the physiology and show its influence even on DNA – the control center within each cell. If the nature of light is still a mystery, the nature of love is even more so. But we do know it makes a difference to another's health if we care for them. It matters to another if we love them.

And it affects our own health too, if we love ourselves. It truly makes a difference to our health to speak a word of love to our feet, our hands, our heart, especially at the end of a busy day.

The Jewish tradition acknowledges this principle. It has developed special prayers of thanksgiving for each of the various apertures of the human body, for their capacity to perform properly the normal bodily functions that we rarely talk about in public conversation. It makes a difference to thank one's eyes, to tell one's sinuses that they did a good job, to speak a word of love to the fingers that performed their intricate tasks with such obedience.

How does this work? Nobody knows. But it has to do with that heart connection, that affinity, that associational link of which the Spindrift people speak.

Norman Cousins, who spent ten years as a communicator and researcher in the medical community, described in *Head First* a research project in the University of California at Los Angeles (UCLA). The immune systems of patients experienced a sharp boost when they were relieved of the depression that followed their diagnosis with life-threatening disease. Cousins told of working with a 29-year-old father suffering massive depression after being diagnosed with multiple sclerosis. Cousins taught the young man Elmer Green's biofeedback technique of "moving his blood around," of holding a thermometer in his hand and using the power of his mind to raise the temperature ten degrees by visualizing the blood flow increasing to his hand. With just this simple demonstration showing him that he had a measure of control over his own body, Cousins helped the young man to reduce his depression and to begin to take an active role in his ultimate return to wellness.

The Mystery of the Body's Capabilities

The body's capabilities to heal itself continue to be a mystery. Studies of less complex life forms remind us of how little we really know.

A. M. Sinyukhin, a biophysicist at Lomonosov University in Moscow, studied the healing process of plants. He cut branches from a series of tomato plants, and then took electrical measurements around the wound as each plant healed. He found a negative current – a stream of electrons – flowing from the wound for the first few days. During the second week, after a callus had formed over the wound and a new branch was beginning to form, the current became stronger, and then reversed its polarity from negative to positive.

For Sinyukhin, the important observation was not the positive or negative nature of the current, but rather the change in its strength. After the polarity shift, as the current strengthened, cells in the area more than doubled their metabolic rate, healing much more quickly.

So he began augmenting the regeneration current using batteries. And after determining the appropriate range of microvoltages, he found that battery-assisted plants restored their lost branches up to three times faster than control plants. He also found that by using current of the opposite polarity, thereby nullifying the plant's own current, he could delay regrowth by two weeks, sometimes three.

To western biologists, this was nonsense. Unexplainable occurrences frighten those who are closed to new ideas, because they undermine their understanding of reality. As one biologist put it,

> *The notion that electricity has anything to do with living things*
> *has absolutely no validity, and any scientific evidence that suggests*
> *otherwise is worthless.*

The Amazing Story of the Newts

The biologist's assertion was made to orthopedic surgeon and researcher, Robert Becker, in response to Becker's application for a small amount of research money for a study of the regenerative capacity of salamanders.

In 1973, Becker's research team began studies toward a better understanding of regrowth in mammals. They examined the effect of direct electrical current on red blood cells in fish, amphibians, reptiles, and birds. The largest red cells they had available belonged to the common green newt. But because a newt is so small, they could not take a blood sample from one of its blood vessels. So they anesthetized the newt and extracted the blood by cutting open its heart, killing it in the process. They took blood from three newts a week.

One day, a member of the team inquired what Becker thought would happen if the wounded hearts were sewn together again. He replied confidently that, like any other animals, the newts would not recover. Becker even checked this conclusion in his standard texts on regeneration which stated that no animal's heart could repair itself if it suffered a major wound. Unlike skeletal muscle, the texts asserted, the heart muscle had no cells waiting that could develop, if needed, into mature heart-muscle cells.

The following week, that team member brought three newts to be used for the blood sample. He announced that they were the same three newts that had been used the week before. They looked perfectly healthy.

Becker immediately anesthetized them, examined their hearts, and found them to be perfectly normal.

Becker had an astounding mystery on his hands. Without delay, he launched a new research inquiry. How could newts survive a massive injury to the heart, yet simply by having their wound sewn up, just one week later their hearts could appear normal again?

He began by ascertaining when blood began flowing again. He found that it started about four hours later.

What Becker and his colleagues observed was considered biologically impossible. As soon as the newt's heart was cut open, blood began pooling around the wound, as expected. It clotted quickly, usually within a minute, sealing the hole. Almost immediately, the nearest red blood cells began breaking open and allowing their nuclei, surrounded by a thin coating of cytoplasm, to move to the injured edge of the heart muscle, guided there by some unknown directive. There they intermixed with the dying and damaged heart-muscle cells and transformed themselves into new heart-muscle cells. Becker described this as unlikely as the engine of a passing car noticing a stranded truck, stopping what it was doing, popping out of the car, rolling itself across the road, climbing under the hood of the truck, and driving off. Those blood cells were actually re-differentiating themselves into new heart-muscle cells. No one considered that to be possible. It had never been seen before.

Meanwhile the newt survived by absorbing dissolved oxygen from the surrounding water through its skin. By the four-hour mark, enough new heart muscle cells were in place for the heart to again begin pumping. Over the next few hours, the process continued, the whole system strengthening and appearing completely repaired after only ten hours.

In *The Body Electric*, Becker asked,

> *Is this fantastic cellular power forever restricted to salamanders,*
> *or does it reside latent within all of us?*
> *Are our systems ready to repair their own damaged human hearts*
> *without transplants or artificial pumps?*

No one has the answers to these questions. It is part of the mystery. But Becker points out that there has never been another regenerative process that has turned out to be forever off limits to mammals.

The Ultimate Mystery

The mystery of life intrigues us. Many think of death as the end of life. But the ultimate mystery, and the subject that never fails to provoke interest, is the question of what happens to our identity at death. Even those who believe that life ends at death will argue their thesis passionately and vociferously.

The Spindrift experiments with bean seeds established, in a laboratory setting, that the identity upon which prayer acts is not limited to an attachment to the physical body, but has an existence of its own. The Bible affirmed this reality long ago. The apostle Paul wrote, in his letter to the Romans:

> *For I am convinced that neither death nor life, nor angels,*
> *nor rulers, nor things present, nor things to come, nor powers,*
> *nor height, nor depth, nor anything else in all creation,*
> *will be able to separate us from the love of God*
> *in Christ Jesus our Lord.* (Romans 8:38)

And Jesus said to his disciples:

> *If I go and prepare a place for you, I will come again and will take*
> *you to myself, so that where I am, there you may be also…Because*
> *I live, you will also live.* (John 14:3, 19b)

The Crucial Question

Whether or not we choose to participate in the mystery of healing depends on our personal response to the question that Albert Einstein asked toward the end of his life, "Is the universe friendly?"

When theologian Karl Barth was challenged to summarize his 12 volumes of systematic theology, he made a simple affirmation in the words of a children's hymn: "*Jesus loves me, this I know.*"

I don't claim any stature like Barth's, but the same conclusion came to me, one night during my studies toward ordination at Emmanuel College, in Toronto. In the darkness, I remember thinking: "Do you believe that God loves you, or do you not? Everything else is interesting, but there is nothing else that really matters." It was my primary "Aha!" moment; my decision to believe it and to trust it has maintained my life of faith ever since.

We Cannot Expect Ever to Know It All

St. Albertus Magnus, a 13th century Dominican theologian, sought, by means of intellect, to "come to know God." At the end of his life, he declared God to be "utterly unknowable apart from what has been revealed in Jesus Christ."

It appears that we can never know it all. The mystery is infinite. But we can still enjoy engaging with it, even as we trust that we exist within its divine loving heart.

Epilogue

Love one another deeply from the heart. (1 Peter 1:22)

In this book, we have offered resource material for beginning and sustaining a ministry of healing, primarily for individuals or groups within the Christian church. We believe it will be useful for anyone who seeks to assist in the healing process of another, in their restoration to well-being.

We three have each taken responsibility for specific aspects of the material, but we all share the book's goals and objectives. We hold in common the view that the foundation of healing is loving – hence the title of this book, *Healing from the Heart.*

We have offered a biblical rationale for the healing ministry and an examination of prayer practices. We have presented specific methods of treatment based on ancient and current bioenergy theories, and referred to contemporary scientific evidence supporting these theories. We have pointed to mysteries and apparent truths which, for some, may challenge our "boggle threshold." In so doing, we acknowledge that creation is far more magnificent than any present understanding, and that divine love remains an unfathomable mystery.

In Jesus, we have all the revelation of truth and love that we need for life. Yet God continues to reveal to us wonders of the universe, even as we live within a limited conceptual framework. New discoveries continue to challenge our present views of reality, both religious and scientific. But as our realization of the wonder of it all is expanded, faith is enhanced.

In all healing, the key consideration must be sincere caring for the individual. We can learn techniques of theories by which we cooperate with the movement of divine power toward healing. And we can develop appropriate healing practices for liturgical use in the church. However, without love we accomplish nothing. Love must be at the heart of it all. As those desiring to grow in the ministry of healing, it is essential that we always make the associational link of love with God through Christ, for it is only the love from the heart of God that heals.

Appendix A

Some Definitions of Healing Modalities

Acupressure is an ancient healing art in which light to medium finger or hand pressure is used at the same points as in acupuncture (see below) to stimulate energy flow.

Acupuncture involves insertion of small needles at points along the meridian lines of the body to activate the flow of the *Qi* or bioenergy. This relieves pain and can increase the immune response by balancing the flow of vital energy throughout the body. As a complete system of healing, it provides effective treatment for numerous conditions, from the common cold and flu, to addiction and chronic fatigue syndrome.

Applied Kinesiology can determine health imbalances in the body's organs and glands by identifying weakness in specific muscles. It studies the activity of muscles and the relation of muscle strength to health, by stimulating or relaxing key muscles. An applied kinesiologist can diagnose and resolve a variety of health problems.

Aromatherapy uses the essential oils extracted from plants and herbs. The therapy is usually administered by massage, in baths, or through inhaling. Aromatherapy is used to treat conditions ranging from infections and skin disorders to immune deficiencies and stress. Essential oils are widely used throughout Europe, and a system of medical Aromatherapy is currently practiced in France.

Bach Flower Remedies are liquid preparations created by immersing flowers in water and exposing these to sunlight or heat. The concept was developed by Dr. Richard Bach in the 1930s to treat specific emotional imbalances. The remedies affect the physical body by stabilizing emotions and balancing negative feelings and stress, thereby removing barriers to recovery and healing.

Craniosacral Therapy manipulates the bones of the skull to treat a range of conditions from headache and ear infections to stroke, spinal cord injury, and cerebral palsy. *Cranio* refers to the cranium, or head, and *sacral* refers to the base of the spine and tailbone.

Healing Touch is an educational program in healing modalities developed for the American Holistic Nurses by nurse Janet Mentgen. This is a worldwide program for the medical community – primarily nurses. It has a clinical focus designed to teach the work of different healers from many different cultures. While it includes the spirituality of the individual, the focus is basically secular.

Recently, due to the large numbers of lay people attracted to the work of healing, the American Holistic Nurses transferred the Certification Process to Healing Touch International in order that lay persons could be eligible for certification. The American Holistic Nurses continue to endorse this program.

Homeopathy derives from the Greek word *homois* meaning "similar," and the word *pathos* meaning "suffering." Homeopathic remedies are "imprints in water" of the vibrational frequencies of natural substances from plants, minerals, and animals. Based on the principle of "like cures like," these remedies specifically match different symptoms and patterns of illness, and act to stimulate the body's natural healing response.

Light and Color Therapy is being investigated in major hospitals and research centers worldwide. Light and color are known to have value as sources of healing. Therapeutic applications indicate that full-spectrum, ultraviolet, colored, and laser light can have value for a range of conditions from chronic pain and depression to immune disorders and cancer.

Magnetic Field Therapy works with the electromagnetic energy patterns within the human body. Magnetic field therapy can be used both in diagnosing and treating physical and emotional disorders. This process has been recognized to relieve symptoms and may, in some cases, retard the cycle of a new disease. Magnets and electromagnetic therapy devices are now being used to eliminate pain, facilitate the healing of broken bones, and counter the effects of stress.

Massage is a system of therapeutic stroking and kneading of the body. The word comes from both the Greek *masso*, to knead, and the Arabic *mass*, to press gently. It fosters a general sense of well-being as well as conditioning muscles and addressing nervous and digestive disorders. There are different styles practiced today. Swedish massage uses a set routine of basic strokes to work over the whole of the body.

Polarity Therapy works through the body's own energy system by placing hands on the body's energy centers and poles to redirect the flow, clearing any energy blocks. The goal is to balance and recharge the flow between positive and negative poles. This causes a calming of nerves, a relaxing of muscles, and an opening of the natural pathways for the healing force in the body to work.

Qi Gong is a system of internal exercise that combines movement, meditation, and breath regulation to enhance the flow of vital energy (Qi) in the body. It also improves blood circulation and immune function. Because Qi Gong can be used by the healthy as well as the severely ill, it is one of the most broadly applicable systems of self-care in the world. In China, it is estimated that 200 million people practice Qi Gong every day.

Reflexology most commonly works with the feet and hands. Working from a map of feet or hands, the reflexologist massages these extremities. The purpose is to send energy signals to stimulate reflex, automatic nerve impulses connected to specific areas of the body.

Reiki is an energy healing system, arising from studies of a Japanese Christian theologian pursuing the particulars of Jesus' laying on of hands. Practitioners are initiated through energy attunement by a Reiki master to channel vital energy. This is done through a light and gentle touching of hands in specific positions on the body.

T'ai Chi is a form of martial art for health based on ancient Chinese ritual dancing. This series of movements and exercises relaxes and balances the body, and serves as a preventative against stress-related disease. The practice involves flowing from one pose into another without a break, thereby expressing the blending of the temporal and eternal.

Therapeutic Touch is a contemporary form of an ancient healing practice in which the practitioner uses the hands as a focus to facilitate healing. The hands are passed through the energy field to assess, clear, and rebalance the field through a consciously directed process of energy exchange. Developed in the early 1970s by nursing instructor Dolores Krieger and noted healer Dora Kunz, Therapeutic Touch is effective in relieving pain, promoting relaxation, and enabling the body to self-heal through the balancing of energies. It is undergirded by a substantial number of master's and doctoral theses, and is now listed in the policies and procedures of many leading hospitals.

Yoga is among the oldest known systems of health and spiritual practice in use in the world today. Research into yoga practices has had a strong impact on the fields of stress reduction, mind/body medicine, and energy medicine. The physical postures, breathing exercises, and meditation practices of yoga have been proven to reduce stress, lower blood pressure, regulate heart rate, and even retard the aging process.

Appendix B

Healing Treatment Techniques

Magnetic Unruffling

Used with permission by Janet Mentgen, RN, CHTP, CHTI, founder of the Healing Touch Certification Program, as published in the *Healing Touch Level 1 Notebook*

"Magnetic Unruffling" is a full-body technique developed by Janet Mentgen to cleanse and clear the complete body, or to remove congested energy and unresolved feelings.

Use: For those with a history of prescription or recreational drug use; also used for those suffering from chronic pain, trauma, environmental sensitivities, systemic disease, or the aftereffects of anesthesia. Useful for emotional clearing.

Procedure:
1. Client lies on the table on his/her back, with shoes and glasses off.
2. After centering and setting intention, healer begins with hands about 12 inches above the head, fingers spread like the prongs of a rake.
3. With one long continuous stroke, pull the hands from the head down the center of the body, to the feet, and off the body. Movement from the head to toes should be in one long slow continuous motion, uninterrupted until coming off the body beyond the toes.
4. If your hands feel as though they have energy accumulating on them, shake them at the end of each pull down the body.

5. Repeat this motion from head to beyond the feet about 30 times or for about 15 minutes, until the energy feels smooth and even, like clear running water.

As an alternative to working down the center of the body, clear one side for about five full passes down the body, then move to the other side of the person's body for five more full passes. Keep moving from side to side in a balanced manner until the whole treatment is complete as mentioned above. If two people work together, one can work on either side. Be sure to work as a team and move at the same pace down the person's body.

Full Body Balance

Adapted from techniques taught by Janet Mentgen and Brugh Joy, MD.

Use: To balance the bioenergy field, to restore the balance of life-force within the body, to restore wholeness, and to re-member the body parts to the whole and to God, through the heart center.

General information about **hand placement** on the body:
This technique connects all the major and minor energy centers of the body and enhances the flow of life force throughout the body. Each of the joints, the soles of the feet, and the palms of the hands easily absorb God's grace, the healing energy. There are also places on the trunk of the body where the energy is absorbed readily. These are major energy centers and places where we naturally place our hands when we are in pain or needing comfort: the lower abdomen, below the belly button, the solar plexus, the center of the chest, the top of the chest at the throat. Hand positions on the head are the brow where anointing occurs, and the top of the head as used in a blessing.

General Instructions:
1. This technique may be done with hands on the body or off. If you are touching the person, always receive permission to touch.
2. Center and allow God's healing energy to flow through you. Your intention is to let this vital energy soak deep into the person's body, filling each cell with God's light and healing power.
3. Spend one to two minutes in each spot, or allow your hands to stay in position until they feel released and ready to move to the next spot.
4. If working with a partner, move to the next position together.
5. Do changes in hand position slowly, gently, and smoothly.

Procedure for working with a partner:

1. Client lies on back with shoes and glasses off, arms at the side, palms down.

2. Stand facing your partner; make connection by placing your palms together. Imagine the light from your spiritual heart centers connecting. Set a common intention.

3. Stand at the feet. Place your hands on (or near) the feet, one hand on the sole of the foot, the other on the top of the foot. If you are physically touching the foot, check to see if the pressure is even and comfortable.

4. Move around to each side of the client. Move the hand from the top of the foot to the ankle, while the hand on the sole of the foot remains.

5. Move the hand from the sole to the ankle, the hand from the ankle to the knee.

6. Move the hand from the ankle to the knee, and the hand from the knee to the hip joint (top of the thigh where the leg joins the pelvis).

7. Move the hand from the knee to the hip, and the hands that were on the hip onto the lower abdomen, below the belly button. (Place hands on the body only with permission.)

8. The hands from the hips move to the lower abdomen. One partner takes a hand from the lower abdomen and places the hand on the solar plexus area. The other partner's hand moves to the center of the chest. The lower body has now been reconnected to the spiritual heart center of the body.

9. Both partners move the hands from the trunk gently and slowly to grasp the hands of the client. Place one hand under the palm; the other hand rests on the top of the client's hand.

10. Move the hand on top to the wrist. The hand connected to the palm remains.

11. Move the hand from the wrist to the elbow, the hand from palm up to the wrist.

12. Move the hand from the elbow to the shoulder, and the hand from the wrist to the elbow.

13. The hands on the shoulder remain. One person now takes the hand from the elbow and places it on the heart center. The other takes the hand from the elbow and places it on the upper chest, close to the neck. Each person will now have a hand on the shoulder and one on the chest and neck.

14. Now move the hand from the shoulders to the brow and crown (top of the head).

15. Ensure your hands feel ready to lift off, then do so gently. Step back, allowing the person receiving to become present, then with your hands 4–6 inches above the body, beginning at the head, slowly brush down the body in one slow steady movement ending 12 inches beyond the feet. Do this three times.

16. End the way you began, connecting with the sole and top of the foot. This helps the person to become fully grounded in the here and now prior to getting up and moving around.

If more than two people assist with this treatment, one person can stand with both hands on the feet through out the treatment and the other person can place both hands on the top of the head while the treatment is being done.

Procedure for Doing a Full Body Balance by Yourself:
1. After centering and setting your intention, stand at the feet with one hand on the sole of each foot.
2. Move around to the right side of the body, and place one hand on the sole of the right foot and the other on the right ankle.
3. Move the hand from the foot to the ankle, the hand from the ankle to the knee.
4. Move the hand from the ankle to the knee, and the hand from the knee to the top of the leg (hip joint, not hip bone).
5. Pause. Repeat on the left leg, beginning with the sole of the foot and the ankle.
6. When both legs have been balanced, place both hands on the hip joints.
7. Leave one hand on the left hip and place the other hand on the lower abdomen, connecting the hip to the pelvis.
8. Leave the hand on the lower abdomen; move the other hand to the right hip.
9. Move the hand from the right hip to the lower abdomen, and the hand from the lower abdomen up to the solar plexus.
10. Move the hand from the lower abdomen to the solar plexus, the hand from the solar plexus to the spiritual heart center. The lower body has now been connected to the heart center.
11. Still standing on the right side, move your hands from the trunk to the right hand, holding the palm and the top of the hand.
12. The hand from the top of the client's hand moves to the wrist.
13. Move the hand from the palm to the wrist, the hand from the wrist to the elbow.
14. Move the hand from the wrist to the elbow, the hand from the elbow to the shoulder.
15. Repeat on the left side.
16. Place both hands on the shoulders.
17. Leave one hand on the right shoulder; move the other hand to the heart center.
18. Leave the hand on the heart center and move the hand from the right shoulder to the left shoulder.

19. Leave the hand on the heart center and move the other hand to the throat area, either at the top of the chest or under the back of the neck.
20. Move the hand from the heart to the top of the chest (throat area), and the other hand to the brow.
21. Move the hand from the throat area to the brow, and the hand from the brow to the crown.
22. To finish, place both hands 4–6 inches above the body. Begin above the head and slowly brush down the body to about 12 inches beyond the feet. Do this three times.
23. Gently hold the client's feet to help him or her come back to the present before getting up.

Procedure for doing the Full Body Balance on Yourself:
This is a wonderful self-care technique, helpful for relaxation. When used at bedtime, it is very helpful in falling asleep. Keep your hands in each position for as long as it feels right or approximately 1–2 minutes. Often when people do this technique on themselves at bedtime, they fall asleep before finishing and then wonder if they should have finished the technique! The healing continues even if you don't finish.

Consider including this prayer when working on yourself:

Gentle loving God, may your light, your love,
and your grace move through me as I pray for the healing
of my body, mind and spirit.
May I let go of that which blocks you finding home in my body;
may I receive deeply all that is offered by you,
as you work to restore me to wholeness and harmony.
I ask for this healing in Christ's name. Amen.

1. Follow the sequence of hand placements outlined above, for a single person doing the Full Body Balance alone.
2. For each hand placement, offer thanks to that part of the body and say the following blessing (or an equivalent): "*May my* (body part) *be filled with God's healing power (or light, love, grace)*". It helps to visualize the body part filling with light; some may experience this as warmth. If you have difficulty reaching your feet, simply imagine that your hands and God's hands are there.
3. Do the right foot, ankle, knee, and hip joint first.
4. Repeat for the left foot, ankle, knee, and hip joint.

5. When your left leg is finished, place your hands on both hips. The hips are big joints and will often absorb a lot of energy so it is useful to spend longer here.
6. Now move both hands to the lower pelvis, one just below the belly button, the other below that hand.
7. The lower hand moves up to the solar plexus area.
8. Again, move the lower hand up to the center of the chest. You have now connected the lower body to the spiritual heart center.
9. The arms are next. Clasp your hands together as in a hand shake, or place them together as in prayer.
10. Move up to hold the wrists, then the elbows, and finally holding the shoulders as in giving yourself a big hug.
11. Once the arms are complete, move one hand to the center of the chest and place the other hand lightly at the throat.
12. Raise the lower hand up to the brow.
13. Finally move the hand at the throat up to the top of the head or crown.
14. Finish with some form of this blessing:

> *May my entire body be filled God's spirit, God's vital living*
> *waters. May I be restored to wholeness and harmony within*
> *myself, within my relationships, and with all of creation.*
> *May the healing power of God present in this clay vessel be used in*
> *God's service. Amen.*

Heart of Christ Connection

A sequence divinely revealed to Rochelle Graham while she was in prayerful contemplation, to bring the high vibration of light and love of Christ into the physical body, the Word incarnate. The inspiration for this body prayer is Ephesians 3:14-21.

Use: This technique for those who are ready to begin a deeper spiritual relationship, for those who perceive themselves as being in a dark time (dark night of the soul), and for those who are ready to move forward on their path of serving God.

Preparation: Begin with the Light of Christ meditation (see Appendix C), asking Christ to be present in your heart. Visualize Christ's presence as light and love; expand that vision to form a chrysalis of light all around you, connecting you to the earth and to the edges of your space.

General Instructions:

The client lies on his/her back with shoes and glasses off. This could be done in a reclining chair if necessary. Do not move to the next position until it feels as though your two hand positions are well connected by the light.

If the client prefers, this sequence can be done with the hands one to four inches off the body.

When people have been previously wounded in the name of Christ, those persons may need to have a blessing used that represents God's light and love with words that suit them and that represent the face of God that comforts them.

Procedure for One Person:

1. Stand on the client's right side.
2. After preparing yourself, ask to connect to the light of Christ in the client's spiritual heart, and place your hand on their heart center. Keep your hand there until the connection feels strong and bright. Imagine a connection between the light in your heart and theirs. The intention is to connect this light and love into their body. Some people may choose to name this as the light and love of God.
3. Place both hands on the client's spiritual heart, in the center of the chest.
4. Leave the left hand on the heart center and move the right hand to the solar plexus. Visualize the light flowing from the heart center to the solar plexus.
5. Move the hand from the heart center to the solar plexus, and the hand from the solar plexus to the lower abdomen.
6. Move the hand from the solar plexus to the lower abdomen, and the hand from the lower abdomen to the left leg at the top of the thigh (the hip joint). This is to connect the spreading of light to the left leg.
7. Keep the hand on the lower abdomen and move the hand from the left hip joint to the right hip joint.
8. Move the hand from the abdomen to the right hip joint; then move the other hand to the right knee.
9. Move the hand from the hip to the knee, and the hand from the knee to the ankle.
10. Move the hand from the knee to the ankle, the hand from the ankle to the sole of the foot.
11. Repeat for the left leg from the hip joint.
12. You have now connected the light and love of Christ through the whole of the body to the legs, the person's means of moving forward in life. Quietly say the following blessing, *"May your steps forward be guided by the light and love of Christ."*
13. Again place both hands on the spiritual heart center of the chest. Take a moment to reconnect to the light and love of Christ.
14. Leaving the right hand on the heart center, move the left hand to the upper chest.

15. Still leaving the right hand on the heart center, move the left hand to the right shoulder.

16. Still leaving the right hand on the heart center, move the left hand back to the upper chest and then to the left shoulder.

17. Leave the left hand on the client's left shoulder. Take the right hand from the heart center and place it on the client's left elbow.

18. Move the hand from the left shoulder to the left elbow, and the other hand to the wrist.

19. Continue the pattern down to include the wrist and hand.

20. Repeat for the right arm and hand.

21. You have now connected the light and love to the person's arms and means of expression. Say the following blessing to them, *"May your voice and expression be guided by the light and love of Christ."*

22. Again place both hands on the spiritual heart center; reconnect to the light and love of Christ.

23. Leave the right hand on the heart center and move the left hand to the top of the chest.

24. Move the hand from the heart center to the top of the chest, and the left hand to the forehead/brow.

25. Move the hand from the chest to the brow, and the left hand to the top of the head.

26. Repeat the following blessing, *"May your thoughts and visions be guided by the light and love of Christ."*

27. Lift your hands off. Remain with the person until they become present. You may want to hold their feet for at least a minute to help them become more present.

Procedure for Working with a Partner:

1. Stand facing your partner, palms connecting with the other person's, and silently prepare using the Light of Christ meditation. (See Appendix C.)

2. Standing on either side of the client, place your hands lightly over the spiritual heart center and ask to connect to the light and love of Christ in their heart center.

3. Each person leaves their upper hand on the heart center and together moves the lower hand to the solar plexus area. The intention is to connect the divine light and love into the next area of the body through both hands.

4. Together move the hands from the heart center to the solar plexus, and the lower hands to the lower abdomen.

5. Together move hands from the solar plexus to the lower abdomen, and place the hands from the lower abdomen on the top of the leg, the hip

joint. The person on the client's right puts a hand on the client's right leg, and the person on the left on the client's left leg.

6. Move hands from the lower abdomen to the top of the leg; move hands from the hip joint to the knee.

7. Move hands from the hip to the knee, and hands on the knee to the ankle.

8. Move the hands from the knee to the ankle, and the hands from the ankle to the sole of the foot.

9. Repeat the prayer, *"May your steps forward be guided by the light and love of Christ."*

10. Both partners again place their hands on the spiritual heart center of the chest and reconnect to the divine light and love.

11. The lower hand stays on the heart center; the upper hand moves to the top of the chest.

12. The hands on the heart center remain, while the upper hands move from the upper chest to each shoulder.

13. Leave the hands on the shoulder while moving hands from the heart center to the elbow.

14. Move hands from the shoulder to the elbow, and from the elbow to the wrist.

15. Move hands on the elbow to the wrist; the hands on the wrist hold a palm of the client's hand.

16. Repeat the blessing, *"May your voice and expression be guided by the light and love of Christ."*

17. Again together, place your hands on the heart center, and reconnect to the divine light and love.

18. Lower hands remain on the heart center; the upper hands move to the upper chest.

19. Move the hands on the heart center to the upper chest; move the hands from the upper chest to the forehead/brow.

20. Move hands from the upper chest to the brow, and hands on the brow to the top of the head.

21. Repeat the blessing, *"May your thoughts and visions be guided by the light and love of Christ."*

22. Remove your hands. Both partners remain with the client until he/she is fully present. Then go to the feet and hold them to assist the person in becoming fully present.

Sacred Cross

This technique was developed by Rochelle Graham in 1995 while working on a client. Her hands were divinely guided in this pattern or sequence; she was then inspired to call it by this name. She also heard words from the Gospel of Thomas: "When the two become one, when you make the inside like the outside, the above like the below, and when you make the male and female one and the same, then you will enter the kingdom of God."

Purpose: This is a sacred technique to connect the client to a very high spiritual vibration and connect this with the physical body.

Use: For people who want to deepen their spiritual connections; for people who are intentional in their spiritual journey. Many practitioners have found this useful in working with the dying. It seems to help them connect with the light of the divine.

General Instructions:

Hold each hand position until the energy between the hands feels balanced and solid. This technique is usually done with the hands touching the person, but if the client is uncomfortable with touching, any or all of the hand positions can be done with the hands off the body.

Procedure for a Single Person:

Notice the pattern of this technique – it repeats a pattern of connecting opposite parts of the body in a cross pattern.

1. After centering and setting your intention, begin by holding both feet, with the thumbs on the sole of the foot and the fingers on the top of the foot.
2. Move around to the right side of the client. Place your hands on the right knee and right ankle.
3. Keep the hand on the right knee, and move the lower hand to the left ankle.
4. Keep the hand on the left ankle, and move the hand from the right knee to the left knee.
5. Keep the upper hand on the left knee, and bring the hand from the left ankle back to the right ankle. You have now completed the first crossover.
6. Move the lower hand from the right ankle to the left knee, and the hand from the left knee up to the right hip.
7. Move the hand from the right hip to the left hip, and the hand from the left knee to the right knee. This is completes the second crossover.
8. Now move the hand from the right knee up to the left hip, while the hand from the left hip crosses over to the right shoulder.
9. The upper hand, on the right shoulder, crosses to the left shoulder; the lower hand crosses to the right hip. This is the third crossover.
10. While one hand remains on the left shoulder, move the hand from the hip up to the spiritual heart center in the center of the chest.
11. The lower hand remains on the heart center and the hand on the left shoulder moves to the right shoulder.

12. Move the hand from the right shoulder to the heart center; move the hand from the heart center down to the solar plexus.
13. The hand sequence now begins to move down the body. The hand on the heart center moves to the solar plexus, and the hand on the solar plexus to the lower abdomen.
14. Move the hand from the solar plexus to the lower abdomen; move the hand from the lower abdomen to the left hip.
15. Leave the hand on the lower abdomen, and move the hand from the left hip to the right hip.
16. Move the hand from the lower abdomen to the right hip, and the hand from the right hip to the right knee.
17. Move the hand from the right hip to the knee, and the hand from the right knee to the right ankle.
18. The hand from the right knee moves to the ankle, while the other hand moves from the ankle to the sole of the right foot.
19. Repeat for the left leg.
20. Holding your hands 6-10 inches from the body, begin above the head gently and slowly brush down the body, including the arms. Do this until the energy feels smooth and still.
21. When the person begins to rouse, hold their feet for a few minutes until they are fully awake and present.

Sacred Chakra Spread

This treatment is based on Isaiah 40:31, *"But those who wait for the Lord shall renew their strength; they shall mount up with wings like eagles."* Janet Mentgen demonstrated it in *Healing Touch, Advanced Practice 1.* Used with permission from J. Mentgen, Founder and Director of the Healing Touch Certification Program, Denver, Colorado.

This technique is a variation of the Chakra Spread taught in Level One of the Healing Touch Certification Program. It is a technique using body prayer (body movements) over the client while also praying a blessing with each movement.

Use: For someone going through a major transition in their life, including assisting a dying person, or during the birth process, or grieving any change or loss. It can simply be used as a profound way to pray over someone in need.

General Instructions:
Begin by asking the person receiving if there is a particular blessing or prayer that they would like said while working. Examples are
  • *May you be filled with the light and love of Christ.*

- *May you be filled with the Holy Spirit.*
- *Peace be with you.*
- *May wisdom fill you and guide you.*

You may choose to prayerfully ask God for a blessing and use whatever blessing comes to you.

Instructions:

All hand movements are slow, gentle, and rhythmic.

1. Begin by holding the sole of the foot with the palm of your hand, with the other hand placed on top of the foot. Hold for at least one minute. Repeat with the other foot. If the person is uncomfortable with feet being touched, hold the hands about an inch from the feet. The intention here is to open the energy flow.

2. Next go to either side of the person and hold the person's hand, with your palm touching the client's palm and your other hand resting on top of the client's hand. Hold the hand for at least one minute. Repeat with the other hand.

3. Without touching the body, move to the head. Ask silently for God's light and love to be present, reach up above the person several feet, and bring the light down forming a column of light, to about 10 inches above the crown. Now gently spread the light to as far as your arms can reach. Say the blessing as you do this. The image is as though you are giving an eagle wings. Repeat this two more times, each time reaching up for the light, bringing it down and gently, slowly spreading the light without touching the body, as you say the blessing.

4. Repeat this "column of light" process three times over each of the following areas: the brow, throat, chest, solar plexus, lower abdomen, top of the thighs, knees and ankles. Each time reach for God's light and gently spread the light over the body while saying the blessing.

5. Without touching the feet, pull the energy off each foot, three times (like pulling off a boot).

6. Return to the crown and repeat the sequence on each area of the body as before, making sure that you spread your arms wide, three times.

7. Repeat this sequence again, completing three entire rounds. Each area will have been blessed nine times.

8. To complete the procedure, return to one hand and grasp it for a moment, as in the opening, mentally connecting with the person, imagining the light from your own heart center connecting with their heart center. Now take the hand resting on top of the client's hand and place it over the center of the chest, the heart center. Remain in this position for as long as it feels appropriate, listening to God's Spirit for guidance when to stop.

9. Release into God's hands with a prayer that the healing continue.

Therapeutic Touch (TT)

Therapeutic Touch is a contemporary interpretation of several ancient healing practices, a consciously directed process of bioenergy exchange during which practitioners use their hands to facilitate healing. The intent is to assist people to repattern their energy in the direction of health. TT can be used alone or with other healing modalities.

Use: Sound scientific research and experience have shown Therapeutic Touch's effectiveness in reduction of pain, promotion of relaxation and sense of well-being, decrease of anxiety, tension and stress, acceleration of wound healing, and facilitation of the body's natural restorative process.

Basic Assumptions:
1. People are energy fields. The bioenergy field is the fundamental unit of the living system.
2. Human beings are bilaterally symmetrical. There is a pattern to the underlying human energy field.
3. Any imbalance in an individual's energy field is a sign of either present disease or potential for future illness or ailment. In illness or injury, the flow of energy is obstructed, disordered and/or depleted.
4. TT practitioners attempt to influence this energy imbalance in order to restore the integrity of the energy "field." Human beings have an inborn tendency towards transformation, transcendence, and improvement of condition. Touching therapeutically is a natural potential in human beings, and can be actualized through the intent to help or heal.

Procedure:
1. Begin by centering. Prepare yourself physically, psychologically and spiritually, connecting within to the Power beyond yourself, and to the inner center of stability.
2. Do an assessment. Use the sensors of the hands to locate asymmetries in the client's energy field. Feelings of difference indicate imbalances or obstructions in the field. These may be experienced by sensations such as heat, cold, tingling, pressure, and congestion. Observation, intuition, and information offered are also considered.
3. Using the motions described in "Magnetic Unruffling" above, make gentle brushes and passes with the hands through the field, down and away from the body. The intention of the mind is to break up areas of hindrance, clear blocks, and assist the free movement of energy throughout the field.

4. Balance the fields. By directing and modulating the bioenergy coming through the practitioner, energies of the client's body are brought into balance. The hands may rest on or near certain areas of the body to facilitate the process.

5. Re-assess and ground the client. Check the field again to assure bilateral balance, and make final adjustments. The client is grounded through the feet.

6. Follow with a ten-minute rest period.

Guidelines for Working With a Group

Sometimes a group of healers will act as unified instruments of God's healing.

Some clients may find a group working together around them overwhelming. Please ask permission for all members to be present. If there are too many for comfort, the others can observe and prayerfully support the healing work.

1. Do a group meditation, centering exercise, or prayer to connect to each other's hearts and to set a joint intention to be instruments of God's healing.

2. Ideally several people would do an assessment and then together share what each noticed. The information of the group helps to create a more accurate picture. Each viewpoint is valid.

3. Together decide on how to proceed. You may choose a technique that two do and the others support, or each of you may be drawn to a specific type of healing. The goal is that you work as a symphony, in harmony rather than discord. Encourage each person to trust that his or her contribution is important to the whole, even if it feels insignificant.

When are two or more better than one?

The combined energy of two or more may assist an individual in releasing long-standing blocks. The energy required to release a block has to be greater than the energy put into storing or avoiding the issue. Therefore the deeper and older the issue, the more support someone will need in healing.

When there needs to be repair to many layers of the bioenergy field following significant trauma (for example, a motor vehicle accident), you will often need four or five partners to work around the person at the edges of the bioenergy field and through all layers.

A team is always useful when there is any concern around discernment, or where there may be concern about boundaries, particularly if the person receiving is of the opposite sex.

Appendix C

Prayer and Meditation Resources

Through prayer, the life of God is nourished in us. The mystic John of the Cross, in speaking of his spiritual journey said to God, *"My soul becomes dry because it forgets to feed on You."* Some ways of prayer may be helpful in feeding the personal spiritual life. These notes were developed by Flora Litt.

Mindful Awareness

Perhaps the most prayerful thing we can do is to "be present" in each moment. It has been said that "life is what happens while we are busy making other plans"! Many of us spend much of our energy on the past or the future, robbing ourselves and others of the blessing of the time that is now.

Therefore, attending to what one is about at any moment – eating, walking, washing dishes, mowing the lawn, conversing, worshipping, or making love – is honoring God's presence in the moment and recognizing the worth of the activity and/or the other in God's sight.

Many persons find the experience of deliberately "walking a labyrinth" an exercise in mindful awareness. This is the ancient practice of walking a laid-out pathway, aware at every step, moving towards the center, and back out again, with spiritual intent.

Noticing God in Daily Life

A further way of prayer in the midst of life is being sensitive to where one's attention is drawn – whether to something in nature or something on a notice board, to an encounter, or to a certain person on the street. One engages in listening prayer by allowing God to speak through these noticings. They may become a metaphor for God's activity in one's inner spirit at that time, or they may draw one to intercessory prayer.

By staying alert to such so-called "coincidences," one will be drawn to prayer and thanksgiving many times during any day, for the Spirit is ever breathing prayer in and through our lives.

In these two ways we can make life a meditation.

Breath Prayer

Ron DelBene, an Episcopalian priest, teaches a simple but effective way of prayer. One gathers in a very few words one's deepest longing, and prays it regularly and intentionally to begin with. Eventually one prays it internally, constantly, and as automatically as breathing.

The prayer has two parts: one's most comfortable and familiar address to God, and one's petition, an asking from the depths of the heart. To open one's deepest heart before God is an act of love and trust. One may continue to use this simply profound prayer for months or longer, and will know when and if it is to be changed. The few words of the prayer are themselves to be prayerfully discerned.

Examples of such prayer might be any of the following. The prayer could also be phrased for another.

- *"Caring God, help me feel your love."*
- *"Mighty God, make me strong in you."*
- *"Lord Jesus, teach me your truth."*
- *"Holy Spirit, guide me in my life."*

Mantric Prayer

A *mantra* is a sound, word, or phrase either spoken aloud or repeated over and over in the mind, voicelessly, to still other activity of the mind and emotion. For the Christian, it helps to bring the attention into the heart, the center of one's being, to commune with God. Ron DelBene's "Breath Prayer" is one type of contemporary mantric prayer.

The Christian roots of mantric prayer go back to the Desert Fathers, and come to us through early Christians, the Russian Orthodox Church, and the Benedictines. The late John Main of the Montreal Priory, in Quebec, taught this practice of prayer to innumerable Christians on this continent and around the world. For a mantra, he used the Aramaic word *Maranatha* meaning "Our Lord, come!" (See 1 Corinthians 16:22b.) One may use this word, saying it slowly in four syllables, "Ma-ra-na-tha." Or one may choose another word such as *Peace, Love, Jesus, Home, Om* or *Soh-hum* (a natural mantra of the breath). These are repeated mentally while breathing normally. Or one may prefer a phrase from a hymn, such as *"Come to my heart Lord Jesus,"* or from the psalms such as, *"Bless the Lord, O my soul,"* or *"The Lord is my shepherd."* Some teachings say that the phrase should ideally be of, but not more than, seven syllables.

To use a mantra, one should enter one's prayer space, and simply begin to repeat the word or words – quietly, gently, and firmly holding the mantra before the mind as a focus. Should the mind wander, or should one cease to repeat the word, one does not berate oneself, but only returns to saying one's sacred word(s). This type of prayer, used twice daily for 20 minutes, brings about profound centering effects and benefits at all levels of being.

Prayer of Examen

Several versions of this type of prayer come from St. Ignatius of Loyola's Prayer Exercises. These include "an examining of consciousness."

Used daily, this type of prayer revisits the day, not to rehearse or rehash its events, but to view once more one's thoughts, words, and actions in the light that the Holy Spirit sheds upon these. It involves first asking for guidance of the Spirit for the grace to see the day and oneself in it as God sees. Then with this assistance, one is drawn to recall where and when God was particularly present and active, and also when and how one was or was not responsive to God's will and leading.

One prays for forgiveness needed, remembers the assurance of God's pardon, and makes whatever resolve for the future to which one is led through the learning. Praise and thanksgiving frame this prayer in its beginning and ending.

The Prayer of Examen brings both the day and oneself to a place of rest, as both are surrendered to God. This prayer need not take a long time, and some people like to journal at the end of it. One can use this type of prayer as a more extended means of "life examen" periodically or when on retreat.

Praying the Scripture (The Lowville Prayer Centre outline)
1. Prepare
- Choose a parable or story easily pictured.
- Settle yourself in a quiet place; quiet yourself.
- Read the selected passage all the way through.
- Ask in prayer for awareness of the presence of the Christ, and for the guidance of the Holy Spirit.
- Read the scripture selection again, attending to the words and phrases you read.

2. Picture
- Read the passage a third time, slowly, sensing your own responses.
- Use God's gift of imagination to picture the passage in detail.
- Be present in the scene yourself.
- Experience the setting. Engage all the senses.
- Feel the emotions.

3. Ponder
- The Latin root is *pondus*, meaning weight. Let the weight of the passage sink deeper and deeper into your being and speak to your heart.
- Ask God to help you to understand the weight of the passage for you.
- Where are you in the scene? Who are you? Do you speak? To whom? Who speaks to you? Touches you? What memory or question is stirred?
- Is there a change in your emotion? Why?
- Take your time. Let your mind be relaxed and open. Listen attentively to any inner speaking.
- Remember that what is given to you now is "the word" for you – today!

4. Promise
- The bridge that connects the time of prayer and daily life involves both awareness and intention. How is God moving in or through you as a result of this meditation?
- Is there a new insight, a new realization of love, of blessing, of encouragement?
- What decision or action are you being led to as a result of this experience?
- What promise do you need to make?

5. Praise
- Praise God for the blessings received.
- Give thanks for the time of being in God's presence.

6. Journal
- Complete the prayer time with a journal entry.

Breathing as Meditation

Much material is available upon the various ways of breathing, but you may begin simply in this manner. Become still in body, sitting upright if possible, spine straight, clothing loose, and begin to notice your breathing. Follow the breath in and out, keeping attention on it.

To enhance the activity, breathe deeply first into the abdomen and then fill your whole being to the slow count of four, holding for the count of two, exhaling slowly to the count of four, emptying your abdomen last and completely, and holding empty for the count of two. Repeat this rhythm over and over for several minutes. The count may be increased (6-3-6-3 or more) as comfortable, but should not be forced. The counting may also be synchronized with your own pulse beat.

Much benefit is effected by the relaxation response. You can engage in this breathing meditation as a prayer of gratitude for the wonderful way in which life energy is renewed.

Since there is a liveliness to the energy *(prana, chi)* being moved or circulated, there may be sensations of heat, light, or vibration during this or any meditation. But we do not judge the effectiveness of the meditation by such sensations, nor intentionally seek them or pay undue attention to them.

Discursive Meditation

The four meditations which follow are examples of discursive meditation. That is, they allow a discourse, an external voice, to guide the imagination.

In discursive meditation, one can not only meditate upon scripture but can also use the imagination in a variety of ways. One common way is to withdraw in the imagination to a peaceful place and rest there, and/or ask awareness of the presence of the Christ meeting one there in some manner.

As well, one can meditate upon dream images or events in the outer life.

Light of Christ Meditation

This meditation was developed by Rochelle Graham, based on Ephesians 3:14-21, where the crucial phrases are, *"that Christ may dwell in your hearts through faith…to know the love of Christ that surpasses knowledge, so that you may be filled with all the fullness of God."*

General Instructions:

This is a useful centering tool to use prior to any healing technique or as a daily routine to help deepen your connection to God.

The term "Christ" in this meditation may have a different meaning for you. It is intended here to be the fire, the flame of the divine within us, the powerful love that transforms (as a fire does) all the spiritual qualities that Jesus embodied. If, as you go into this meditation, Christ is represented to you in another form, simply go with what is presented by the Spirit.

This meditation may be done with your eyes open or closed. Seat yourself comfortably, feet uncrossed and touching the floor, arms and shoulders relaxed.

Meditation:

1. Begin by noticing the sensations in your body, especially noting your feet and their connection to the ground.
2. Become aware of your breath. Allow your breath to move deeply into your being. With each breath in allow your focus to go deeper into your being. As you breathe out, let go of any distractions.
3. Now take your awareness to the center of your chest and look deep within to your spiritual center. Ask that the light and love of Christ be present there in your heart. If at first you don't notice or feel anything, ask for the sensation to be stronger. If you still have no sensations, continue anyway, trusting that this is unfolding as it needs to.
4. Connect to the divine light and love. You may feel it as warmth or you may see it as a flame. For some it may take the form of the sun or a star. Invite that light and love to expand and fill your entire being. Just as the sun shines unconditionally on all of the earth, so does this light of Christ want to shine on all parts of your being.
5. Let it fill your physical body, flowing through all parts right down to fill your feet. Let this root and ground you. It may even flow through your feet into the earth.
6. With each breath in, allow it to flow further into your body, filling and nourishing each cell.
7. Now imagine the light, shining from the core of your being, sending light and love beyond your physical body to shine in all directions just like the sun. Just as the sun gives unconditionally, so let this light shine.
8. Invite it to form a chrysalis or cocoon of light and love all around you. Ask this light to be in balance above and below, side to side, and front and back.
9. From this place of being filled and grounded with the light and love of Christ, state your intention to be an instrument of healing for the highest good. (If you are doing laying on of hands, you would place your hands on the person now.)
10. After sitting quietly in this for a few moments, gently bring your awareness back to your physical body and then back to the room.
11. If you are doing this as a daily meditation, slowly build up the time you spend in this form of visual prayer.

Option for a Group:

Gather in a circle. Begin as described above. Once the intention has been stated, ask participants to let the rivers of light or living water (John 7:37-38) flow from their heart to the person on their right. Also ask them to be open to receive this light and love of Christ from the person on the left.

This may also be used for Intercessory prayer. Invite everyone to face their palms into the center of the circle and then place the names of individuals in need of healing in the circle. Invite the circle participants to allow the light and love from their hearts to flow to those named. Close with a prayer releasing those named into the hands of God.

Tree of Life Meditation

This meditation, also from Rochelle Graham, was inspired by references in Revelation 22:2, and Genesis 2:9 to the "tree of life."

General instructions:

This can be a very useful visualization/meditation to help you ground and center quickly. This meditation may be done with your eyes open or closed.

Make yourself comfortable, feet uncrossed and touching the floor, arms and shoulders relaxed.

If the images presented here are not working for you, allow God to present images that may work. The theme is to connect to all the sources of God's energy available through the earth and heaven.

Meditation:

1. Begin by noticing the sensations in your body and especially noting your feet and their connection to the ground.
2. Become aware of your breath. With each breath in allow your focus to go deeper into your being. As you breathe out, let go of any distractions.
3. Invite a tree to come into your mind. It may be a tree you are familiar with, it may be a tree that your mind gives you.
4. Observe the tree. Notice as many details as you are able – its size, whether it is alone or with other trees. Notice the season. Listen to any sounds, and smell the air.
5. Now move closer to the tree until you are close enough to merge with the tree. Either imagine that you are the tree, or imagine what the tree feels like.
6. Take your awareness down the inside of the trunk into the roots. Follow the roots into the ground, noticing how deep they go. Feel the soil. Are there rocks, or sand, or rich fertile humus?
7. Like the tree, allow all that the earth has to offer you to flow up into the roots. It may be water, minerals, or vital energy from the earth. Allow yourself to be nourished completely, and like the tree allow this nourishment to flow all the way up the trunk. This is God's gift from the earth.

8. With each breath allow the energy to flow higher and higher up the trunk, filling the branches right to the tips of the tree. Feel all of you being nurtured by the energy of the earth.
9. From the tips of the branches allow the light of God (or sun, or whatever else in the sky is helpful) to flow in, again filling and nourishing the tree.
10. Allow this energy to flow downward this time, right down to the roots. Slowly as it moves down, feel the tree filling with this light until every fine hair of the roots is also filled.
11. When you are connected to the divine above and the earth below, when you are rooted and grounded and connected to the love of God, state your intention within yourself to be an instrument of healing and peace.
12. Now slowly disconnect from the tree and become aware of your own body, notice how you feel. Notice your feet, your arms. When ready bring yourself back to the present and look around.

Green Pastures and Waters of Rest Meditation

Based upon Psalm 23:1-3b, this meditation by Flora Litt may be read slowly, quietly yet distinctly, to another or to a group, with appropriate pauses for imaging. Or it may be read in its entirety by an individual onto an audio tape, and then played as a personal meditation. Timing is very important. Read each sentence slowly, calmly, with plenty of time to allow images to build in the mind.

Preparation for group or individual meditation (these instructions may be read):
1. Become comfortable in your chair, feet flat on the floor, back straight, and hands resting in your lap. Or lie on your back, spine straight, with hands at your sides. Close your eyes.
2. Relax the body with a few deep breaths, breathing from the abdomen. If any particular area is tense, breathe directly into that area and release the tension with each exhalation until it feels cleared.
3. Allow your mind also to become still and quiet, as if a gentle breeze has blown away all busy or anxious thoughts, leaving only a sense of calm mental space.

Meditation:

When the group (or individual) feels settled, proceed with the following guided meditation.

Into the open space in your mind, a pastoral scene arises – a field where white, golden-hearted daisies dance, where purple-headed clovers nod, and green grasses bend and stretch in a gentle breeze.

Be present there with all your senses keenly aware. See the summer scene. Hear the birds and insects. Feel the sun's warmth and smell the fragrances.

You notice that a stream is not far away, and you hear the soft murmuring of its flowing waters. You are drawn toward it as if led by an unseen hand.

On its grassy bank, beside a leafy tree, you sink down to rest, suddenly realizing the weariness within you. Lying back on the moist, warm earth, you feel gratitude for its supporting strength and allow God's earth energies to soak into your being. Your heart draws in the vibrant green of the grass upon which you lie and of the leafy branches overhead.

Then, in a clear but quiet voice, words come to your inner ear – "I am your Good Shepherd. You shall not want for anything you need. I bring you to green pastures and lead you beside waters of rest, that the life in you may be restored. I do this for I am Jesus, and I love you."

The profound love in these words washes away the weariness of body and soul. You feel fresh and clean. It is as if you had been washed in the waters of the stream.

You rest in this refreshing love, listening to the softly singing waters of the stream, knowing that the life in you is being restored.

Arising at last, you are drawn to scoop up the clear, cool water of the stream. You kneel. Cupping water in your hands, you drink deeply. Then, as you gaze once more upon the scene, a prayer of responsive love and gratitude stirs within you. You know you will remember this place, the words and the water, and the One who met you there. You know you can return whenever you need, and find refreshment for the living of your life and your service for Jesus in the world.

Slowly, you turn away. You notice you are smiling, and your step reveals the renewed vitality within you.

In your mind, return to the room in which you are. Move your hands and feet a little. Open your eyes when you are ready, becoming aware of your familiar surroundings.

The Potter and the Clay Meditation

Flora Litt based this meditation upon Jeremiah 18:1-6. It may be read slowly, quietly yet distinctly, to another or to a group, with suitable pauses for imaging. Or it may be read in its entirety by an individual onto an audio tape and then played as a personal meditation. Timing is very important. Read each sentence slowly, calmly, with plenty of time to allow images to build in the mind.

Preparation for group or individual meditation (these instructions may be read):
1. Become comfortable in your chair, feet flat on the floor, back straight, and hands resting in your lap. Or lie on your back, spine straight, with hands at your sides. Close your eyes.
2. Relax the body with a few deep breaths, breathing from the abdomen. If any particular area is tense, breathe directly into that area and release the tension with each exhalation until it feels cleared.
3. Allow your mind also to become still and quiet, as if a gentle breeze has blown away all busy or anxious thoughts, leaving only a sense of calm mental space.

Meditation:

When all appear to be relaxed and settled, or when one's own body and mind are relaxed and receptive, continue with the following guided meditation.

You find yourself alone in a potter's shop. See the many pots and jars of various sizes and shapes: some painted brightly and some not; some newly shaped and waiting to be fired, and some darkened with age; some perfect and some flawed. But each has its place. Smell the faint odor of dust in the air, and hear a rhythmic whir coming from an inner room. The potter must be at work.

You approach the door of the inner room. Looking in, you see the potter at the wheel. A nod of the potter's head invites you to enter. You watch in silence as the potter, with skillful hands, perfects a clay vessel. How beautiful it is! What symmetry and balance in the graceful curves!

Your thoughts go round and round with the turning of the wheel. "Would that I could be so perfect!" you say to yourself. "But I am not. I know I am not. I am like one of those flawed ones in the shop," you say to yourself. And you recognize that you feel sad about this.

Then you see that the potter has finished the vessel being worked upon and laid it aside, taking instead another from a nearby shelf. It's an off-shaped pot with a crack in its side. You watch the pot being broken by hands that seem both strong and gentle, capable and purposeful. The pieces of clay are moistened in water, then gathered up firmly in the potter's hands.

You talk with the potter, asking what has caused the difficulty. You are told that there can be many reasons: mishandling by a helper, an accident, too fast or too slow drying, many different reasons. But, you are told this pot is still valuable, and thoroughly redeemable. You believe this as before your eyes the clay is drawn together and placed again upon the potter's wheel. You see it being remolded, becoming a new creation.

As you watch, you want to become like that vessel. You want to offer yourself into the hands of the original potter, God, who understands what has happened, and who knows exactly what is needed to make you into a new creation.

As the wheel before you whirls, you close your eyes and surrender yourself into God's kind and loving hands, trusting that as you become soft and pliable, you will be reshaped as God intends and become again the way God has always seen you – beautiful, perfect, without flaw. The old creation is being transformed. You rest in God's hands, as surrendered clay.

You are drawn from your reverie. The wheel has stopped. This potter has finished the work. With a nod of satisfaction, the potter gently places the re-formed vessel upon the drying shelf.

You express your thanks to the potter, and breathing a prayer of thanksgiving to the Great Potter of your life, you slowly return to the room in which you are now.

Open your eyes as you are ready. Take your journal and draw or write of this experience.

Retreat

To go on a prayer retreat is a practice more familiar to Roman Catholics than to Protestants, but today many of all faiths and no faith are rediscovering the benefit of "coming apart" before they "fall apart." For the Christian, a retreat is a means of change from the daily round, a time to rest, pray, talk, listen to God, and enjoy communion with God. More and more persons in all denominations are searching out and experiencing the enrichment of prayer life through retreat.

One can move into retreating slowly and by stages. Some people approach silence and solitude more easily than others. It is very helpful to have the assistance of a person trained as a Spiritual Guide. Retreat Centers usually can provide such assistance.

Appendix D

Healing Service Resources

Healing service notes

The following notes have been prepared by Wayne Irwin and printed in various bulletins for services of healing. Excerpts from these may be useful in providing information and inspiration for persons in the congregation as they come to the service of prayer for healing, and for reflection at home.

Notes #1

Jesus healed. He healed as a sign of the in-breaking of the reign of God, and he healed because he cared. Healing was essential to his ministry. The church, also, is given the gift and responsibility for healing. In the early church, anointing, the laying on of hands with prayer, exorcism and the visitation and communion of the sick were regular and important elements of ministry.

Unfortunately, during the Middle Ages, the liturgical actions of anointing and communion of the sick became almost exclusively associated with the dying (extreme unction and viaticum). These practices were opposed by most Reformers and a liturgical ministry with the sick did not become part of the Reformed tradition. Although services for the visitation and communion of the sick continued in Anglican practice (and Wesley included communion of the sick in his "Sunday Service of the Methodist Church in North America") the emphasis was on sickness as testing of faith or punishment for sin.

By the late 19th century, Reformed understandings were changing. *Eucticologion* (1867), the first Presbyterian service book since the *Westminster Directory*, included a service for the visitation of the sick. The Canadian Presbyterian *Book of Common Order* (1922) followed *Eucticologion's* lead. The 1932 United Church of Canada *Book of Common Order* included a service of communion with the sick.

But no such service was included in the 1969 *Service Book*. It was believed that ministry with the sick lay in medical missions and in ministries of counseling. In 1977, however, the United Church's committee on Christian Faith produced the booklet, *A Christian Perspective on Healing*. It was a call not only for ministries of healing based on medical and psychological models, but for a careful liturgical ministry with the sick: "...Christian healing involves the trust that God works through dimensions of reality which we cannot understand to bring healing and health."

This dimension of healing is represented through symbols which point to God's working and love: prayer, laying on of hands, touch, anointing with oil, etc. These symbols are genuine instruments of healing, and should be so used in the church's ministry of healing alongside normal medical procedures. They open us to a power which medical science alone does not possess. To this end it is important that services and resources be made available so that the church can respond appropriately when there is a desire for some liturgical action which will express our trust in the presence and love of God with a sick person.

Notes #2

Services of healing have a biblical heritage appropriate for the full life of the church. Anointing and the laying on of hands are acts closely related to the covenant of faithful love between God and Israel, and between God and the church. In scripture, monarchs are anointed, prophets commissioned, the Holy Spirit conferred, the sick healed, and the dead raised in acts of faith accompanied by anointing with oil, the laying on of hands, or touch in another form. The symbolism of touch has survived almost universally among churches in the laying on of hands at baptism, confirmation, and ordination. And the power of touch is finding renewed acceptance as is the unity of the whole person.

In the New Testament, faith, forgiveness of sins, and healing are frequently inseparable but distinct aspects of one experience. Out of compassion and mercy, God works to bring about reconciliation that restores peace between God and humanity, among individuals and communities, within each person, and between humankind and the creation. Guilt, anxiety, fear, broken relationships, and the loneliness of alienation all contribute to human sickness. Healing, in the Christian sense, is the reintegration of body, mind, emotions, and spirit that permits people, in community, to live life fully in a creation honored by prudent and respectful use.

In our healing service, four themes are intertwined: God's word, growth in faith, forgiveness of sin, and human touch.

In scripture, God's word reassures us of the creator's love and compassion. Jesus' acts of healing, the healing ministry of the New Testament church, and contemporary experiences of healing all testify to the health and fullness God makes possible in human life.

Faith in the inclusive sense of trust and belief in God's unmerited goodness is an integral cornerstone of the New Testament understanding of healing. Individuals and communities of believers nurture each other in their mutual growth in faith. God does not promise that we will be spared suffering, but does promise to be with us in our suffering. Trusting that promise, we are enabled to bear the unbearable and recognize God's sustaining nearness in pain, in sickness, and in injury.

Forgiveness of sin often is closely linked with healing in the New Testament. The connection of forgiveness and healing affirms the psychosomatic unity of individuals that is recognized by modern health sciences. It admits the importance of openness and honesty to every relationship of love. It sets health in the context of relationships restored by confession and forgiveness.

In the New Testament, touch plays a central role in the healing ministry. The power of touch is recognized, whether in the anointing with oil, the laying on of hands, or less formal gestures of holding someone's hand or touching a wound. Jesus frequently touched others: blessing children, washing feet, healing injuries or disease, and raising people from death. Jesus also allowed himself to be touched, washed, embraced, anointed. To allow oneself to be touched is an act of openness. To touch another is an act of acceptance in which a person transfers something of oneself to another: love, affection, protection, strength, power, acceptance. Touch in the healing ministry embodies the embrace of God for the redeemed creation when, in the mystery of last things, God will "make all things new."

Orders of Service

Services may be reproduced for use in one congregation or group with acknowledgment.

Service of Healing (Congregation)

The following service has been regularly used by the Lowville Prayer Centre. It was prepared by Wayne Irwin.

(* People standing, if able)

GATHERING FOR WORSHIP
As you enter the sanctuary, please observe silence that all may be assisted in preparing.

PRAYER FOR PREPARATION (for private personal use)
> *Eternal God, prepare me to receive your grace.*
> *Prepare my mind to hear your word.*
> *Prepare my heart to open to your love.*
> *Prepare my will to respond to your appeal,*
> *through the power of your Spirit,*
> *and in the name of Christ.*

SILENT ACKNOWLEDGMENT OF GOD'S PRESENCE

PRAYER OF APPROACH
One: O God, to be turned from you, is to fall,
           to be turned to you, is to rise,
           And to stand in you, is to abide forever.
Many: Grant us in all our duties, your help,
           in all our perplexities, your guidance,
           in all our dangers, your protection,
           and in all our sorrows, your peace;
           through Jesus Christ our Savior.

*HYMN

CONFESSION
One: It is the caring activity of Christ that cleanses us from all that is past.
           It is the acknowledgment of our need that prepares us for the grace to
           be received.
           Let us, therefore, confess together:
All: Understanding God, your desire revealed in Christ
           is to prosper us and not to harm us,
           to renew us in your love and to give us hope.
One: We recognize before you that in things we have both done and left
           undone,

we have sometimes turned our back upon your love,
and that sometimes, our relationship with you has been disrupted
by experiences we did not choose.

All: But, we have made choices that have contributed to pain,
made decisions that only you can fully understand.
And so we ask that you heal our relationship with you.
Release us from all that keeps us in fear and shame
and help us sense your leading in our living
towards the day of our full delight within your will,
and the life of joy in journeying in your way,
through Jesus, the Christ, our Savior and Redeemer.

SILENCE FOR PERSONAL CONFESSION AND FORGIVENESS OF OTHERS

REMEMBRANCE OF GOD'S MERCY

One: God is merciful.

Many: Christ is merciful.

All: God is merciful.

*ASSURANCE OF PARDON

One: Hear the Good News of the Gospel!
There is no longer any condemnation for those who live the love of
Christ,
because it is that love which sets us free from the bondage
of self-condemnation and the fear of death.

Many: In Christ, we are assured that God forgives us,
and invites us to attend the heavenly banquet.

*ACCEPTANCE OF THE GOSPEL

One: Do you believe God's good news?

Many: We do.

One: Praise be to God!

*RESPONSE OF PRAISE (Tune: Old 100th)

> *Praise for your wondrous works of pow'r,*
> *Praise for your tender cov'nant love,*
> *Praise for the whisper of your voice,*
> *Your word of healing in our life.*

*EXCHANGE OF PEACE

Many: The peace of Christ.

SERVICE OF THE WORD

PRAYER FOR ILLUMINATION
Many: Amen.
READINGS IN HOLY SCRIPTURE
Lector: This is the word of God!
All: Thanks be to God!
SERMON

SERVICE OF COMMUNION AND HEALING PRAYER

THE OFFERING OF INVITATION
INTIMATION AND INSTRUCTION
PRAYER FOR GUIDANCE
Many: Amen.

THE OFFERING OF GIFTS
(Symbolized by bread & wine, anointing oil, and money)
* PRESENTATION OF THE OFFERING (Tune: Franconia)

These gifts we offer now,
in honor of your Name.
Receive these symbols of your Life
and bless us with the Same.

BLESSING OF THE ANOINTING OIL
One: Gracious God, you anointed Jesus of Nazareth with your Holy Spirit
        and with power to bring to everyone the blessings
        of life lived in divine relationship with you.
Many: Praise belongs to you, O God!
One: Connect the benefit of your Holy Spirit's presence
        with the imposition of this oil, O God,
        that those receiving this anointing may in faith be restored and made
        whole,
        that the lives of all those in weakness may be transformed by the risen
        Christ.
Many: Glory belongs to you, O God!
One: Anoint your church, also, we pray, with this same Holy Benefit,
        that all who share in the sufferings of Christ may also know Christ's
        victory,

and be enabled to witness to the gospel of healing and wholeness,
through Jesus, the Christ, our Savior.

Many: Praise and glory belong to you, O God!

PRAYER OF HUMBLE ACCESS

One: We do not presume to come to your Table, O merciful God,
trusting in our own righteousness, but in your great mercy.

Many: Our worthiness is your gift to us,
your gift of grace, your gift of love;
and you are God, the Divine Giver.
Grant us therefore Precious One, so to partake of your Life,
that our bodies and souls may be restored,
that we may henceforth recognize your protection,
and trust the constancy of your provision.

THE GREAT THANKSGIVING

One: God is with you.

Many: And also with you.

One: Lift up your hearts.

Many: We lift them up to our God.

One: Let us give thanks to God.

Many: It is right to give God thanks and praise.

One: It is indeed right that we should praise you, gracious God, for you
created all things.
You formed us in your own image: male and female you created us.

Many: When we turned away from you in sin, you did not cease to care for us,
but opened a path of salvation for all people.

One: Therefore, with your servants and prophets, and with all your saints
of every age,
we give thanks and raise our voices to proclaim the glory of your name.

All: Holy, holy, holy God, Creator and Ruler of all,
heaven and earth are full of your glory.
Hosanna in the highest!
Blessed is the One who comes in your name, O God.
Hosanna in the highest!

One: Holy God, source of life and goodness, all creation rightly gives you praise.
In the fullness of time, you sent Jesus, the Christ, to share our human nature,
to live and die as one of us, to reconcile the world to you.

Many: Praise be to you, O God.

One: On the night of betrayal unto death, Jesus took bread;
          and after giving thanks to you, broke it, gave it to his disciples, and said,
          "Take, eat; this is my body which is given for you.
          Do this for the remembrance of me."
          After supper Jesus took the cup of wine;
          and after giving thanks, gave it to them,
          and said, "Drink this, all of you: it represents the new covenant,
          sealed by my death, the guarantee that you are forgiven.
          Whenever you drink of this cup, do it for the remembrance of me."

Many: Thanks be to you, O God.

One: Gracious God, by the death of Christ you have destroyed the power of death,
          and by raising Christ to life you have ordained for us
          eternal life forevermore.
          Therefore we proclaim the mystery of faith.

All: Christ has died;
          Christ is risen;
          Christ will come again.

One: Recalling the death of Christ, proclaiming the resurrection,
          and looking for the coming again in glory,
          we offer you, O God, this bread and this cup.

Many: Send your Holy Spirit upon us and upon these gifts,
          that all who eat and drink at this table may be one body and one holy people,
          a living sacrifice in Jesus, the Christ.

All: Through Christ, with Christ, and in Christ, in the unity of the Holy Spirit,
          all glory is yours, God most holy, now and forever.

THE LORD'S PRAYER (Ecumenical version)
          Our Father in heaven, hallowed be your name,
          your kingdom come, your will be done, on earth as in heaven.
          Give us today our daily bread.
          Forgive us our sins as we forgive those who sin against us.
          Save us from the time of trial, and deliver us from evil.
          For the kingdom, the power, and the glory are yours, now and forever.

SYMBOLIC ACTION
The form of "Intinction" is used (bread dipped in grape juice).

Sharing the Symbols of Christ

One: Jesus Christ, the bread of heaven.

Many: Amen.

One: Jesus Christ, the cup of salvation.

Many: Amen.

Anointing and Laying on of Hands

Those desiring prayer for self or another are invited to remain at the kneeler.

Other Prayers for Healing

One: For (name), O God, you hear our prayer.

Many: And you answer in your love.

Commendation

One: Now we commend these our concerns… for each other… and ourselves… into the safekeeping of the Christ.

Many: Help, save, strengthen, and defend us, O God, by your grace.

Words of Testimony

As applicable.

GOING FORTH

*Hymn

*Benediction

One: We have come to God for the forgiveness of sin,
        for the strengthening of faith,
        for the restoration to wholeness
        of body, mind, spirit and emotion.
        Our relationship with God and with the world has indeed been healed.
        Let us go forth empowered to serve and glorify God all our days,
        by the power of the Spirit at work within us,
        through the Christ, our Healer and our Redeemer.

Many: God blesses us and keeps us.
        God's face shines upon us.
        God looks upon us with favor
        and gives us the Peace of Christ.
        Thanks be to God!

Fellowship

Service at the time of Anointing (Group)

Bruce McIntyre, minister of Carstairs United Church, has been engaged in a ministry of healing prayer in his congregation for many years. A "Healing Room" has been established in the church, and persons come by appointment during the week for Healing Touch. This is the liturgy used at the time of anointing:

Leader: The Rite of Anointing presents us with a means of experiencing the compassion and the love of our heavenly Father. The sacrament is meant to lead us into an ever deepening awareness of God's presence in our lives as we turn to the source of all life. God is now present among us and desires to be intimately involved in every aspect of our search for wholeness.

God patiently waits to be invited into our lives. God never disregards our free will, but gives us the freedom to accept or reject the grace that he provides for us.

The first requirement for receiving the Lord's healing love is to ask God to assume dominion over our entire being. We need to recognize any futile attempts on our part to earn salvation through self-effort and return to the foot of the cross where the ransom was paid once and for all for every one of us.

It is important for us to invite the risen Jesus Christ into our life. The risen Jesus Christ is aware of our needs and is longing to draw us closer to himself, but we must take his nail-scarred hand.

READING: a lesson of Jesus healing.

PRAYER:

Together: Loving God, we realize that there are areas in our lives where we need your healing touch. We have hesitated to ask for healing for a variety of reasons, but we come to you today, feeling somewhat like the person in the scripture that we just read. Amen.

Leader: We have come together in the name of our Lord Jesus Christ, who restored the sick to health, and who himself suffered so much for our sake. The risen Jesus Christ is among us as we recall the words of the Apostle James: "Is there anyone sick among you? Let him call for the elders of the Church, and let them pray over him and anoint him in the name of the Lord. This prayer, made in faith, will save the sick person. The Lord will restore his health, and if he has committed any sins, they will be forgiven."

We entrust our sick (brother or sister) (name) to the grace and power of the Risen Jesus Christ, that the Lord may ease (his or her) suffering and grant (name) health and salvation.

Leader: Let us pray.

Lord God, all-comforting Father, you brought healing to the sick through your Son Jesus Christ. Hear us as we pray to you in faith, and send your Holy Spirit, the comforter from heaven, upon the holy oil, which nature has provided to serve the needs of people. May your blessing come upon all who are anointed with this oil, that they may be freed from pain, illness, and disease and made well again in body, mind, and soul.

May this oil, which you have blessed for our use, bring the healing that you have for our loved one (name).

In the name of our Lord Jesus Christ we pray.

(Anoint each person's forehead and hands.)

PRAYER OF ANOINTING:

I anoint you to be healed by God through Christ's gift of the Holy Spirit.

I anoint your hands to be the blessed hands of Christ that will share the gift of God's holy healing presence. In the name of the Father, the Son, and the Holy Spirit.

(After the laying on of hands, close with the Lord's Prayer for protection.)

Anointing Liturgy for a Group in an Informal Setting
prepared by Flora Litt

(It is suggested that the group be seated in a circle formation, with a low table in the center. Two leaders will be needed; they should speak from within the circle until the actual time of anointing. On the appropriately draped table, there should be a Christ candle and an earthen pot of about 4–6 inches in diameter, containing oil to a depth of two inches. The oil may be inexpensive cooking oil, or olive oil, with no more than a drop or two of fragrant oil in it. A small pot with the anointing oil is placed beside the candle. A double sheet of paper towel should be placed on the floor under each chair. Following the anointing, hands may be laid on any who are sick, and who so desire, by the leaders who will pray over them. Meditative instrumental music may be played as the group gathers. No bulletin is necessary.)

LIGHTING OF CHRIST CANDLE

Leader 1 (standing): Let us stand together. We light this candle as a symbol of the presence of the living Christ in our midst, and we greet those around us with the words, "Christ is with you," responding with "And also with you."

People respond as indicated.

Leader 1 (seated): We gather in Christian community as friends, to offer support to one another, and especially to those among us who are sick and in need of the healing touch of Jesus. This blessing we ask for them, and pray for ourselves also, renewal of the spiritual energy which manifests in healing for body, mind, emotions, and relationships. We trust that God is with us, even when we and those we love are hurting. We believe that God desires to touch us in love and bring us to wholeness. This is our faith as we prepare to receive the blessing of anointing.

Let us pray in silence, acknowledging personal need, or the need of another, and expressing love and thanksgiving for what God is willing and able to do.

MEDITATION

Leader 2: Amen.

What is it about oil, that we should use it to express God's goodness, love and healing? You are invited now to experience the oil through your senses and your imagination, both of these in themselves gifts of God. Come forward one by one to the table.

(Leader 2 moves to the center to demonstrate.)

Dip the fingers of one hand into the oil, and grasp that hand in the palm of the other hand in this manner, and then return to your seat with oil in hand. Someone will come to any in the circle who find it difficult to move.

(Leader 2 returns to the circle. Music may be softly played during this time, and during the following meditation. When all have touched the oil, Leader 2 continues, speaking slowly and meditatively, but with a clearly audible voice.)

Leader 2: Look at the oil in your palm. Notice its texture and its fragrance. Begin to work it into your hands, spreading it along your fingers and onto the backs of your hands. Do this slowly and notice the feeling in your hands as you gently but firmly massage the oil in. Feel its goodness. When you have finished massaging, bring your hands to rest on your lap, using the paper towel from the floor under your seat, if need be, for them to rest upon. Have your hands in an open position. Allow your whole body to become still and at rest. Close your eyes and slowly take a few deep breaths in and out, breathing in the Spirit-breath of

God with every inhalation, and breathing out any physical or emotional tension of which you become aware. Allow yourself to become deeply quiet, letting go of all anxious thoughts, seeing them carried away on the wind of the Spirit. Rest in silence for a few moments.

(SILENCE *for not more than one minute*)

Leader 2 *(continues)*: Now, keeping your eyes closed, imagine yourself walking toward a place in which you are relaxed and feel safe. It may be in a setting in nature, or a certain place in your home – wherever you feel comfortable. You see the place now not far from you, and you are slowly walking toward it, noticing as you go the colors, sounds, and smells, and your feelings. As you get closer you are aware of things in greater detail, and you enjoy the sensations of the place.

You want to find a place to rest, and you look around. Finding a place to which you are attracted, you move toward it and settle yourself there. You know you are completely alone in this place. Then you notice a large earthen jar close beside you. It is filled with oil much like you massaged your hands with earlier. You put both hands into this jar of oil and feel its smooth, soothing quality. Taking handfuls of the oil you let it drip through your fingers. Scooping it up, you rub it on your arms and legs, and the back of your neck, your forehead and your chest. Feel the oil flowing over your whole body; breathe deeply of the oil's aroma as it enfolds you. Feel the oil and the aroma seeping into you, touching you wherever there is hurt, within or without, with healing and with peace. If there is any special place in you still in need, apply more oil in that place, lovingly and gently, giving thanks for its cleansing, soothing, and restorative qualities.

Feeling much strengthened, you rise up, stretching your body and your arms upward in praise to God, the Creator of oil and the Giver of its blessing. You slowly leave your resting place, and begin to make your way back to this room, arriving when you are ready. Keeping your eyes closed, feel yourself present here with the group.

(While the people are still in this experience, one or more of the following passages of scripture may be read with silences between.)

Leader 2: Let us hear the words of scripture:

Psalm 133

> *How very good and pleasant it is when kindred live together in*
> *unity! It is like the precious oil on the head,*
> *running down upon the beard, on the beard of Aaron,*
> *running down over the collar of his robes.*

It is like the dew of Hermon, which falls on the mountains of Zion.
For there the LORD ordained his blessing, life forevermore.

SILENCE
Luke 10:30, 33-35

Jesus said, "A man was going down from Jerusalem to Jericho,
and fell into the hands of robbers, who stripped him, beat him,
and went away, leaving him half dead...

A Samaritan while traveling came near him;
and when he saw him, he was moved with pity.
He went to him and bandaged his wounds,
having poured oil and wine on them.
Then he put him on his own animal,
brought him to an inn, and took care of him."

SILENCE
James 5:14-15

Are any among you sick? They should call for the elders of the
church and have them pray over them,
anointing them with oil in the name of the Lord.
The prayer of faith will save the sick, and the Lord will raise them
up; and anyone who has committed sins will be forgiven.

Leader 2: Bless these readings to our understanding, O God. Amen.

Leader 1: Let us praise the God of goodness and healing, responding at each
pause with the words, "Blessed be God." And let us pray blessing
upon the oil for anointing.
  We praise you, God, Creator of all creatures and of this substance,
oil. Out of the great silence of your love has come forth your Word,
Jesus the Christ, to live among us, to die and be resurrected for us,
that we might be brought to the wholeness of salvation.

All: Blessed be God.

Leader 1: We praise you, Lord Jesus, that through your human life you have
come to know the afflictions of our humanity, and desiring to minister healing to us you touch us in your great love.

All: Blessed be God.

Leader 1: We praise you, Holy Spirit, who breathes life into us afresh in the anointing with oil, that we may be free of all dis-ease of spirit, mind, heart or body.

All: Blessed be God.

Leader 1: And now, O God, may your blessing come upon this oil, symbol of your healing love. May its touch upon us be the sign of your forgiveness of all our sins, your deliverance from all that would depress or oppress us, and your restoration of our complete being into wholeness. In the loving and powerful name of Jesus we pray.

All: Amen.

ANOINTING

Leader 1: You are invited to come forward in groups of four to six persons, to stand around the table for anointing. You will be anointed on your forehead and the palms of your hands. When all in the first group have been anointed, the next group should come, and so on. At the conclusion, any who have not been able to come forward should raise a hand for anointing where they are seated.

(Music may be played if desired, as the following words are spoken over each person during their anointing on forehead and on the palms of the hands. Leader 1 anoints and speaks words such as the following.)

Leader 1: I anoint you in the name of God, your Creator; Jesus Christ, your Healer; and the Holy Spirit, your Sanctifier. May God's grace and peace be upon you and within you. Amen.

(When all have been anointed, an invitation may be given to those who desire further prayer and the laying on of hands. This will be done by the leaders together, with spontaneous prayer being offered.)

PRAYERS OF THANKSGIVING AND INTERCESSION

(Leader 1 invites the group to offer prayers in spoken word or in silence, concluding the prayer time by saying the Lord's Prayer in unison.)

SENDING FORTH AND BENEDICTION

Leader 1: As you have received Christ Jesus the Lord (in anointing with oil, and the laying on of hands), continue to live your lives in him, rooted and built up in him and established in faith, just as you were taught, abounding in thanksgiving (Colossians 2:6-7). And may the blessing of God continue with you always. Amen.

Service for the Elderly, of Anointing and Laying on of Hands
prepared by Flora Litt

(This service is intended to minister specifically to the elderly within the Christian community, and may be held in the church, in an individual family home, or in a hospital, nursing home, or other long-term care facility. It recognizes that while many of the elderly enjoy good health into advanced years, others experience the physical, mental and emotional pain of debilitating infirmities, with probable attendant limitation, fragmentation, or separation. This anointing seeks the healing of the whole person: spirit, mind, emotions, body, and relationships. It is meant to be communal, with family members, friends, and caregivers invited to attend and participate in the liturgy. The service need not be somber, and may include a celebration of Holy Communion. If it does not include the Eucharist, then the service may be conducted throughout by lay persons. There is no need of a bulletin, and the people may simply be invited to respond with "Thanks be to God" following the scripture readings, and with "Amen" following the prayers.)

OPENING WORDS

Leader: The love and fellowship of God are with us here, as we gather for a celebration of our life in Christ Jesus, and for the anointing with oil and the laying on of hands for healing into wholeness.

Hear the words of Jesus:

Come to me, all you that are weary and carrying heavy burdens,
and I will give you rest. Take my yoke upon you,
and learn from me; for I am gentle and humble in heart,
and you will find rest for your souls. For my yoke is easy,
and my burden is light. (Matthew 11:28-30)

HYMN OF PRAISE *(Optional)*

PRAYER OF CONFESSION

Leader: Gracious God, we confess our sins before you. We confess our failure to give you heartfelt thanks for the blessings of our lives, for the joys and the sorrows, for all the ways you have guided, supported and strengthened us in times of trouble and weakness. We confess the doubts and fears that even now threaten to undermine faith in your constancy and provision. Forgive us for all our words or actions that have failed to show through us the nature of Jesus to others. It is in his name that we pray,

People: Amen.

ASSURANCE OF PARDON

Leader: God does not hold our sins against us, but forgives us all that is past. Our sins are blotted out; God remembers them no more. We are assured that in Christ Jesus we are forgiven and freed from all guilt!

People: Thanks be to God!

SERVICE OF HOLY COMMUNION *(Optional)*

PRAYERS OF THANKSGIVING AND PETITION

Leader: Let us pray. We give you thanks, O God, for your presence, your power, and your everlasting love. We give you special thanks this day for the witness of faith of the elderly among us. We are blessed with the joy of their friendship, the companionship of their lives, and the example of their obedience to you. We pray that through the anointing and laying on of hands today, they may be strengthened to continue to witness the saving power of your Son's death and resurrection which heals us and draws us to you. Prepare us who are to give and receive this ministry, and open us now to hear your word through scripture. In the name of the risen Christ we pray,

People: Amen.

(One of the readings to follow may be done by a family member, or friend.)
First reading: 1 Peter 1:3-9
Leader: This is a word of living hope.
People: Thanks be to God!

MEDITATIVE HYMN *(Sung or played on tape)*

Second Reading: Matthew 5:1-10
Leader: This is the word of Christ Jesus.
People: Thanks be to God!

LEADER'S WORDS FOR MEDITATION

(A very brief homily may be given on this passage. Poverty of spirit, gentleness, patience, mercy, etc. may be especially evidenced in the lives of the elderly as their identification with the suffering of Christ has become more visible in their lives. As children of God, we all come to God with childlikeness, openness and simplicity. We trust that God who has blessed us all the days of our lives, continues to bless us with the fruit of the Spirit abiding within us in love and power, and strengthens us for the living out of these in our relationships.)

INVITATION

(The Leader will alter the invitation such that it is suitable for the situation.)
Following our prayer, let those who desire anointing and laying on of hands for renewing of strength and healing into wholeness, come forward one by one if able, or be brought by another, or remain in their seat for ministry to be received by indicating their desire in the raising of a hand or nodding of their head.

PRAYER BEFORE ANOINTING

Leader: Let us pray. O God, you are a strong tower to all who put their trust in you. Grant to these who now receive anointing, deliverance from all dis-ease of body, mind, or spirit. In your love, and by the power of your Holy Spirit, touch them with your healing, and restore them to the wholeness of everlasting life in you. In Christ's name we pray.

People: Amen.

(As each one receives anointing and the laying on of hands, words such as the following may be spoken.)

Leader: (Name), you are anointed in the name of God, Father, Son, and Holy Spirit, and as these hands are laid upon you, may our Lord Jesus minister the blessing of healing to you, that restored to balance of spirit, soul, and body you may rejoice in wholeness, and be at peace in Christ's love. Amen.

(At the conclusion of the ministry, the leader may extend arms toward all in blessing.)

Leader: Let us pray in the words of the Psalmist:

> *God, you taught me when I was young, and I am still proclaiming*
> *your marvels. Now that I am old and gray, God, do not desert me;*
> *let me live to tell the rising generations about your strength and*
> *power, about your heavenly righteousness.*
> (Psalm 71:17-19 Jerusalem Bible)

People: Amen.

CLOSING HYMN

BENEDICTION

Leader: The love of God enfolds us, the peace of Christ fills us, and the companionship of the Holy Spirit remains with us always.

People: Amen.

Family Anointing Service

Notes: One or two family members should prepare a worship center including a candle and matches, Bible, glass bottle containing the oil. The oil for anointing may have been blessed at a regular healing service, or may be blessed in the family with the use of the prayer suggested. The roles of "One" and "Another" may be taken by any child able to read or by an adult.

One: We light this candle to remember that the Spirit of Jesus is here with us. We come together to celebrate our life as a family, to give thanks to God for one another, and to pray for one another, asking God's blessing and wholeness for each.

Song: "God Is So Good...God's So Good To Me." *(one verse only)*

One: I know God is good to me because _____ *(gives a simple, short answer as a model for others in the family).*
All sing verse again.
Another: I know God is good to me because _____ .
(Follow the pattern of singing and response until all members of the family have had opportunity to participate.)

One: Loving God, we thank you for all your goodness to us, and for our life together.
Family: Amen.

Song: "Thank You, God, for Giving Us Life" *(or other thanksgiving song or hymn known to the family)*

One: As we join our hands, let us pray together, asking God to help us. Caring God, we want to forgive one another as you forgive us.
Family: Help us, God. *(response after each petition)*
One: We want to love one another as you love us.
Family: Help us, God.
One: We want to care for one another and for others as you care for us.
Family: Help us, God.
One: We want to be healthy, as you intend for us to be.
Family: Help us, God.
One: We pray in the name of Jesus, who showed us how to forgive and love and care, and who taught us a prayer to say together, "Our Father..." Amen.

One: Let us show our love as we give a hug to each other.

Another:When we look at this oil we think of the gift oil is to us in our human
            life: oil from seeds and plants for cooking and eating, for healing the
            body, and for the pleasure of perfumes, oil from the earth for light
            and fire to warm us.

Family: Thank you God for the gift of oil.

Another: *(lifts up the bottle of oil and holds it)* This oil is special. We place it
            upon one another's forehead and hands to remind us that the Holy
            Spirit is a gift to each one, blessing us with God's love, warmth, light,
            and health (or healing).

*(Or pray as follows: "God, bless this oil, that as it is placed upon the forehead and
hands of each one, we are reminded that the Holy Spirit…")*

Another: *(turns to the nearest family member, dips a fingertip in the oil, makes a
            sign of the cross on the forehead and touches the palm of each hand,
            saying)* God blesses you in love.

*(The oil is then passed to that person who anoints the next family member nearest,
until all are anointed and the oil is returned to the table.)*

One: God has blessed us in love that we may in turn love others, and show
            our love in what we think and say and do. Let us pray for God's bless-
            ing of love and care for others as we say their names as a prayer to
            God for each one. *(Space is allowed for the offering of names.)*

One: Listening God, we leave these ones in your care, and we thank you for
            hearing our prayer, in Jesus' name.

Family: Amen.

Song: "Alleluia, Alleluia, Give Thanks to the Risen Christ" or "Jesus Loves
            Me" *(or other song or hymn of praise known to the family)*

One: Let us join our hands. Let us be happy in remembering God is with us
            and within us always, helping us to live in love.

Family: Amen.

Covenanting Service for Healing Teams

OPENING PRAYER HYMN: "In Loving Partnership We Come" verses 1 and 2
(Strathdee)

Leader: The church recognizes the diverse gifts of its members, and celebrates
the particular ministry of each person. There are different kinds of
spiritual gifts, but the same Spirit gives them.
People: There are different ways of serving, but the same God is served.
Leader: Christ is like a single body which has many parts.
People: All of us are Christ's body, and each one is a part of it.

Addressing the congregation (if congregation present)
Leader: These persons have been called by God to serve among us, in the ministry of Christian healing, within and beyond this congregation. They
have accepted their call, and are before us as witness of their willingness to serve.

Addressing the healing team (if the congregation is not present)
Leader: You have been called by God to serve in the ministry of Christian
healing. You have accepted your call, and now express your willingness to serve, as the Spirit enables you.

Leader: Sisters and brothers in Christ,
having prayerfully considered the calling and responsibilities of
your ministry, are you prepared to serve in Christ's name and for
the glory of God?
Healing team members *(answering individually)*:
I am.
Leader: Do you promise to exercise your ministry faithfully, showing forth
the love of Christ?
Healing team members *(answering individually)*:
I do, relying on Christ's grace.

(If the congregation is present)
Leader: Members of the congregation,
you have heard the promises of our brothers and sisters in Christ,
who have answered God's call to service. Let us affirm our intention
to live in covenant with them.

People: We celebrate our partnership with you in the service of Jesus Christ. We promise to love you, honor your healing ministry, and support you with prayer and encouragement, that together we may be a faithful church of Jesus Christ.

(If the congregation is not present, move directly to the anointing and laying on of hands.)

Leader: Anointing, with the laying on of hands, is a symbolic act, whereby the church in every age recognizes God's call to ministry in the lives of faithful men and women, and asks the Holy Spirit to confer on them the gifts of ministry.
(touching the head, the heart, and the palm of each hand)
        (Name), I anoint you in the name of Christ, for the exercise of your healing ministry, by the power of the Spirit.
Person: Amen.
Leader: These hands are laid upon you that the Holy Spirit may fill, strengthen, and equip you with every good gift to do God's will, in the name of Christ.
Person: Amen.

Leader: Let us pray.
        Loving God, we thank you for these persons who have responded to your call for ministry. Let your blessing rest upon them in fullness, as they are entrusted with the exercise of Christian healing. May the love of Jesus permeate their heart and flow from them as living waters.
People: Amen.

Closing hymn prayer: "In Loving Partnership We Come" verses 3 and 4

Appendix E

Music Resources

The following hymns are listed as suggestions for use in services of healing. Following each hymn is the name of the text author and composer (author/composer) and a designation as to whether the hymn is in the public domain (PD) or is controlled by a copyright holder (three-letter code).

All the suggestions that are not in the public domain are covered by **LicenSing, Copyright Cleared Music for Churches**. If you have a license with *LicenSing*, you are free to copy the words to all the suggestions listed. If you do not have a license with *LicenSing* and you wish to copy words of songs that are covered by copyright, you have one of two options:
1. Obtain a *LicenSing* license by contacting Wood Lake Books, Inc. at 1-800-663-2775 (in Canada) or Logos Productions, Inc. at 1-800-328-0200 (in the United States).
2. Obtain permission from the individual copyright holders. The copyright holders, represented by a three-letter code, are listed below.

CCC	Common Cup Company	1-604-931-4683
HOP	Hope Publishing Company	1-800-323-1049
KLU	Klusmeier, Ron	1-250-954-1785
LAN	Lankshear-Smith, Doreen	1-807-557-3345
MCD	McDade, Carolyn	1-508-349-2283
OCP	Oregon Catholic Press	1-503-281-1191
SAM	Sam, Jeeva	1-306-545-2511

SEL	Selah Publishing	1-914-338-2816
SFA	Songs for a Gospel People	1-800-663-2775
STR	Strathdee, Jim & Jean	1-916-481-2999
WIL	Willow Connection	011-612-9948-3957
WOG	Word of God	1-313-677-6490
WPP	Weston Priory	1-802-824-3573

Hymns

A Woman in the Crowd (Wren/Hopson) .... HOP
All the Way My Savior Leads Me (Crosby/Lowry) .... PD
Amazing Grace (Newton/Excell) .... PD
As Comes the Breath of Spring (Ritchie/Dale) .... PD
Ask Me What Great Thing (tr. Kennedy/Malan) .... PD
Breathe on Me, Breath of God (Hatch/Jackson) .... PD
Christ is Alive (Wren/Williams) .... HOP
Come and Find the Quiet Center (Murray/attr. White) .... HOP
Creating God Your Fingers Trace (Rowthorn/Haydn) .... HOP
For the Healing of the Nations (Kaan/Purcell) .... HOP
From You All Skill (Kingsley) .... PD
God, Whose Almighty Word (Marriott/Giardini) .... PD
God Whose Giving Knows No Ending (Edwards/Perry) .... HOP
Great Is Thy Faithfulness (Chisholm/Runyan) .... HOP
Hark, the Glad Sound (Doddridge/ad. Webbe) .... PD
Here I Am, Lord (Schutte) .... OCP
Hope of the World (Harkness/Genevan Psalter) .... HOP
How Sweet the Name (Newton/Reinagle) .... PD
In Loving Partnership (Strathdee) .... STR
Jesus' Hands Were Kind (Cropper) .... HOP
Jesus, Keep Me Near (Crosby/Doane) .... PD
Jesus, Lover of My Soul (Wesley/Perry) .... PD
Jesus Heard with Deep Compassion (Patterson) .... HOP
Jesus Stand Among Us (Pennefather/Filitz) .... HOP
Like the Murmur (Daw, Jr./Cutts) .... HOP
Long before the Night (This ancient love) (McDade) .... MCD
Now Thank We All Our God (tr. Winkworth/Cruger) .... PD
O Changeless Christ (Dudley-Smith/Turle) .... HOP
O Christ the Healer (Green) .... HOP
O for a Thousand Tongues (Wesley/ad. Mason) .... PD
O God beyond All Praising (Perry/Holst) .... HOP

O God of Every Nation (Reid, Jr.) .... HOP
O Holy Spirit, Enter In (tr. Winkworth/Nicolai) .... PD
On Jordan's Bank (tr. Chandler/arr. Havergal) .... PD
Open My Eyes That I May See (Scott) .... PD
Praise to the Lord, All of You (Klusmeier) .... KLU
Sing Praises to God Who Reigns (tr. Cox) .... PD
Songs of Thankfulness (Wordsworth/Hintze) .... PD
Spirit Divine, Attend Our Prayers (Reed/Cruger) .... PD
Spirit of God, Descend upon My Heart (Croly/Atkinson) .... PD
The Head That Once Was Crowned (Kelly/Clarke) .... PD
The King of Love My Shepherd (Baker) .... PD
The Lord's My Shepherd (Scottish Psalter) .... PD
There is One Lord (Alstott) .... OCP
There's a Wideness (Faber/Steiner) .... PD
Thou Whose Almighty Word (Marriott/Giardini) .... PD
Touch the Earth (Murray/Gibson) .... HOP
We Are One (Lankshear-Smith/Sam) .... LAN/SAM
When Jesus the Healer Passed through (Smith) .... HOP
Will You Come and See the Light (Wren) .... HOP
Within a Womb of Darkness (Patterson) .... HOP
Word of God, Come Down on Earth (Quinn) .... SEL
Your Hand, O God (Plumptre) .... HOP
Your Hands, O Christ (Plumptre; rev. Hobbs) .... SFA

Choruses and Songs

A Light Is Gleaming (Good) .... HOP
Alleluia, Alleluia, Give Thanks to the Risen Christ (Fishel) .... WOG
Christ Is Risen (anon/Hasidic folk melody) .... PD
Come Drink Deep (McDade) .... MCD
Drink Living Water (Fulmer/Zaragoza) .... OCP
Flow River Flow (Hurd) .... OCP
Hark, the Herald Angels (Wesley/Mendelssohn) .... PD
Heal Me (Watts) .... WIL
Heal Me, O God (Norbet) .... WPP
I Am the Light of the World (Strathdee) .... STR
I See a New Heaven (McDade) .... MCD
In the Morning (Norbett) .... WPP
Lay Your Hands Gently (Landry) .... OCP
Love Calls Me Back (Bates) .... WIL

Appendix F

Stories from Congregations

West Point Grey United Church

Vancouver, British Columbia

West Point Grey United Church is situated in the west side of Vancouver, near the University of British Columbia. Because of its proximity to the University, the congregation usually has a significant percentage of academically inclined people, both faculty and students. Many retired ministers also call this church home. Therefore, the faith of this congregation is strong, but scientific reasoning and a rational approach are important. They also have had a strong social justice and pastoral care component in their outreach ministry.

In the fall of 1995, three women (Margaret Berthelson, Joyce Brown, and Phyllis Bernez) who had experienced Healing Touch decided they would like to offer a workshop on healing in their congregation. The congregation could see the application of hands on healing work in pastoral care.

They met with their Christian Education worker and with the minister of the church, Rev. Cheryl Black. They received support from these two important players and got a "go-ahead" for a workshop in January 1996. This ten-hour workshop taught the spiritual and scriptural roots of healing, the basics of the laying on of hands, as well as other simple techniques. The intent of the workshop was to explore the concepts of being a healing presence, and to learn how to allow God's gift of healing to come through.

The workshop was repeated six months later, for a second group.

Practice Sessions

Out of these two workshops came a committed group of individuals who decided to meet biweekly to practice. They were fortunate to have a volunteer, Ginny Mulhall, who was more experienced in healing work, as their mentor. Ginny attended the practice sessions to guide the group.

The practice sessions began with the group sitting in a circle. They were led in a centering meditation to help them come to a peaceful place after their busy days and to help them prepare for healing work. They then decided on a specific technique to practice, and moved to treatment tables to do this work. The advantage of tables over chairs is that the receiver is able to relax easier while lying down. Each person had an opportunity to receive a treatment and to practice giving.

They then debriefed the experience and learned from each other. The group had a closing circle, holding hands.

The Fruits of Their Labor

"All these events made us a feel a spirit was at work...a movement was growing. We felt we were being given a direction," Joyce said. The practice sessions were important in confidence building. Now the group was ready to present this ministry to the congregation and community.

The opportunity came very soon. For Maundy Thursday of 1996, the Minister and Worship Committee decided on a "Healing Offering." Following a short service, those attending were invited to the adjoining gymnasium where there were chairs, tables, and a circle for "foot washing." As the tables were filled, Healing Touch was also offered to those who were sitting. It was a remarkable "servant offering," and was remembered by some long after the event.

That was the formal introduction to the larger community. Following that, one practice session a month was opened for those who wanted to receive healing.

Since then, there have been requests from within the congregation and from other congregations, from people who would like to receive support and comfort through the gifts of healing.

One story is particularly worth noting. A request for support came from a woman in the congregation who was widely known in the church, deeply loved and respected. She had just been diagnosed with extensive inoperable cancer. The "Healing Group" was ready to be of service. Except for Saturdays, which were kept as family days, two women went every day from mid-July to mid-November, just before this wonderful woman died.

While it was hard for this group of dedicated caregivers to accept that healing in this case did not mean physical cure, they were aware of the tremendous healing that did happen.

What this group has found essential in developing a healing ministry:

1. A minister who is supportive.
2. A designated coordinator who receives the request, who calls and schedules healing sessions.
3. The importance of always going out in pairs to provide mutual support.
4. An experienced mentor who is willing to work with the group providing guidance and support. This can be managed by telephone if there is not someone local.
5. A group based and well-grounded in a church committee. This particular group comes under the guidance of Pastoral Care.
6. An ongoing invitation to people to come to the group to share, to learn, or to receive.

Walton Memorial United Church
Oakville, Ontario

Early in 1996 the Official Board of Walton Memorial United Church in Oakville, Ontario, supported 18 members of the congregation in their vision to begin a Service of Prayer for Healing. The idea for these services did not come as a sudden vision; the group had been building toward this for quite some time.

It began several years earlier with the start of a prayer group and a prayer chain. Members of these groups also participated for the next four years in Weeks of Guided Prayer – retreats in the midst of life – held in their church.

Members from these groups then began to do a study on healing and wholeness. This study allowed them time to discern both the need for this service within the church and their own personal call to this ministry. With the support of their minister, Rev. Jim Gill, and the congregation, members of Lowville Prayer Centre were invited to provide training and to assist with the first services. This gave the group time to grow in courage, confidence, and experience, as they stepped out in faith, developing this new ministry.

They report that it is amazing to look back over the time since then to see how these 18 people have discerned their call, whether as pray-ers, ushers, or coffee hosts. Their original lack of confidence and feelings of unworthiness appear to have been transformed as they stand faithfully at each service before God and his people, to pray with the help of the Holy Spirit for the needs of others. The Healing Ministry Team has grown spiritually, learned a greater trust in God's love and power, and developed a greater sense of fellowship with each other. They find it a great privilege to pray for others, and acknowledge that God has truly blessed them in their efforts to be a blessing to others.

Carstairs United Church
Carstairs, Alberta

Bruce McIntyre, minister at Carstairs United Church, tells this story of a healing experience in the Philippines.

In 1980, I, along with a group from Canada, went for 20 days to one of the reputable healing centers in the Philippines. The group included ten people from our United Church congregation (Carstairs United Church), my wife and one of our sons.

A service of worship, similar to our Sunday morning service, was held at the beginning of each day. Each morning there was a class on holistic healing. Part of each afternoon was spent in the healing room.

I found the morning classes to be very similar to the course "Holistic Approach to Health and Disease" which I had taken from the Rev. Bob Keck (the author of *The Spirit of Synergy*) in 1977 and 1978 in Crystal Lake, Illinois. In fact, when the healing instructor in the Philippines had to be away for three days, I taught the three morning classes, using my notes and experience with Bob Keck.

I taught the basic concepts of energy fields and holistic healing; awareness of altered states of consciousness, and how to consciously alter our own state of consciousness by meditative prayer; and the importance of being guided by the presence of the Holy Spirit.

In the afternoon, the group was divided into three time periods to go to the healing room. As each group entered the waiting room we were asked to fill out a request form for healing. As we waited for our turn to go into the healing room, the group sang a song or mantra in Pilipino calling on the Spirit of God's healing to flow through the healing teams.

I was allowed to be an observer in the healing room (only if I had permission from the person who was receiving the healing). The work in the healing room was conducted by teams of two or three Filipinos. There was a Filipino medical doctor present.

The people who came into the healing room removed their outer clothing and then lay on one of the four tables. They were covered with a sheet. One of the teams of healers at each table read the healing request, then uncovered that part of the body requiring healing and worked directly on that area of the body. The healing team manipulated the area. In some cases it looked like they actually opened up the area and removed or manipulated the area beneath the skin.

After the healing session, the person's time was their own to enjoy the beautiful countryside. It was necessary for most people to visit the healing room more than once.

In the evening, a man by the name of Rustico, who was an electrician in charge of maintenance from a downtown hotel, came. People could have him come to their room to have him do healing on them. I was asked to be the contact person for Rustico. I would take the request of the person and then go with Rustico to each room and witness his work. He would lay hands on and pray.

A few days before we left, he blessed each one of my fingers and hands, and had me lay hands on people who were requesting healing. Rustico also taught me how to relieve a headache by touch. I have learned as much from Rustico as I have from anyone else.

Some people came home disappointed. One woman died of cancer while we were there. But one man from our congregation who hadn't been able to breathe through his nose since serving in the war came home breathing normally, and continued to do so. On our way home, during a stopover in Manila, one woman, who could only see shadows, suddenly exclaimed, as she looked down from the mezzanine of the hotel, "I can see goldfish swimming in the pond!" One man from Calgary, who as a result of a back injury had not been able to bend over, excitedly shared with everyone, "See, I can touch my toes!"

Even though people from our congregation came home excited about their healing experiences, people who had not been there remained skeptical about the obvious healings that had taken place.

St. Andrew and St. David United Church
St. John, New Brunswick

Chris McMullen has written that when he was called to the Church of Saint Andrew & Saint David, one of the things the congregation sought from his ministry was "an interest in healing ministry."

Shortly after he arrived, the Session committed the church to developing a ministry of prayer for healing. They compared it to having a choir; every church wants to have a choir, although not everyone wants to be a member of it. In the same way, they felt that the ministry of prayers for healing should be an essential element of a church and its ministry, even though not everyone would participate.

They have been sponsoring workshops in healing twice a year, attended by persons from their own and other congregations. They have been hosting "services of prayer for healing" once a month, on a weeknight in an intimate chapel, and once a quarter in the sanctuary with a more formal order of service. At these services, persons may receive anointing with oil, and prayer with laying on of hands from teams of three trained intercessors.

In addition to these corporate expressions, there has been a ministry of telephone intercession. Chris, as minister, has used anointing with oil and the laying on of hands in counseling or pastoral visiting as appropriate. It is not unusual to see a small group praying with someone after church, with the laying on of hands, often right in the coffee lounge. The rest of the congregation is comfortable with this, although many would not participate in the circles themselves.

Trinity United Church
Lively, Ontario

In the monthly Sunday morning Communion services in Trinity United, in Lively, prayers for healing have been "built in." The Session approved it, and the congregation has responded with enthusiasm.

Persons come forward, or "process," to receive the elements. There are two stations available for worshippers to receive the bread and the grape juice. A third station has been established, which persons can subsequently attend if they desire prayer for healing for themselves or for others. About a quarter of the congregation regularly avail themselves of the benefit of this option.

As minister Thom Davies explains, "So as not to embarrass the introverts among us, the congregation sings the repetitive Taizé chorus, 'Eat this bread, drink this cup,' throughout."

Two persons serve at each station, including the station for prayer. As each person is anointed, these words are used: "I anoint you in the name of Jesus Christ." As hands are laid on, these words are spoken: "May the compassion of God, which is present here with us now, enter your mind, your body and your spirit, and heal you from all that would harm you."

Appendix G

Primary Principles for a Healing Ministry

1. God is over and in all creation. God is transcendent, the Creative Power of the universe, beyond conceptualization and beyond all names. But God is also immanent as the Divine Presence, made known to us through the incarnation of the Christ in Jesus of Nazareth.

2. We and all creation are meant to share in God's shalom. In Hebrew "shalom" means to be whole, to be sound, to be safe, to be in peace.

3. Human beings are a created unity of body, mind and spirit, and are interconnected with one another.

4. As essentially spiritual beings, creatures made in the image of God, we are subject in this earthly dimension to experience the tension between good and evil, and the effects of imperfect choices and responses.

5. Healing as restoration to wholeness and balance is the will of God.

6. The church is called by Jesus to continue the ministry of healing.

7. The church is empowered by the Holy Spirit, and equipped for the fulfillment of this calling.

8. The compassion of Christ mediated through the loving heart of an ordinary Christian is the agency of healing.

Bibliography

Abrams, Jeremiah and Connie Zweig, eds. *Meeting the Shadow*. Los Angeles:
    Jeremy P. Tarcher, 1991.

Achterberg, J. *Imagery in Healing: Shamanism & Modern Medicine*. Boston: Shambhala, 1985.

Barnstone, Willis, ed. *The Other Bible*. San Francisco: HarperCollins, 1984.

Barrow, John D. *Theories of Everything: The Quest for Ultimate Explanation*.
    Oxford: Oxford, 1991.

Bateson, Gregory. *Mind and Nature: A Necessary Unity*. New York: E. P. Dutton, 1979.

Becker, Robert & Gary Selden. *The Body Electric: Electromagnetism and the
    Foundation of Life*. New York: Wm. Morrow, 1985.

Benor, Daniel. *Healing Research: Volumes 1 and 2*. United Kingdom: Helix Editions Ltd., 1993, 1994.

Benson, Herbert. *The Mind/Body Effect*. New York: Simon & Schuster, 1979.

——. *The Relaxation Response*. (Avenal, NJ: Outlet Books, 1990)

——. *Timeless Healing: The Power and Biology of Belief*. New York: Scribner, 1996.

Bentov, Itzhak. *Stalking the Wild Pendulum*. Rochester, VT: Destiny Books, 1988.

Bird, Christopher & Peter Tompkins. *The Secret Life of Plants*. New York: Avon, 1972.

Bliss, Shepherd, ed. *The New Holistic Health Book*. New York: Viking Penguin, 1985.

Bohm, David. *Wholeness and the Implicate Order*. New York: Routledge, 1980.

Borg, Marcus J. *Meeting Jesus Again for the First Time*. New York: HarperSanFrancisco, 1994.

——. *The God We Never Knew*. New York: HarperSanFrancisco, 1996.

Borysenko, Joan. *Minding the Body, Mending the Mind*. Don Mills: Addison-Wesley, 1987.

Brennan, Barbara A. *Hands of Light*. New York: Bantam, 1988.

Burton Goldberg Group, Comp. *Alternative Medicine: The Definitive Guide*. Fife, Washington:
    Future Medicine Publishing, 1995.

Capacchione, Lucia. *The Picture of Health*. Santa Monica, CA: Hay House, 1990.

——. *The Power of Your Other Hand*. North Hollywood, CA: Newcastle, 1988.

Capra, Fritjof. *The Turning Point*. New York: Bantam, 1982.

——. *The Web of Life*. New York: Anchor, 1996.

Casey, Juliana. *Food for the Journey: Theological Foundation of the Catholic Health Care Ministry*. St.
    Louis, MO, and Washington, DC: Catholic Health Association of the United States, 1990.

Cassell, Eric J. *The Nature of Suffering and the Goals of Medicine.* New York: Oxford, 1991.

Casti. John. *Searching for Certainty: How Scientists Predict the Future.* New York: Wm. Morrow, 1990.

Chopra, Deepak. *Ageless Body, Timeless Mind.* New York: Harmony Books, 1993.

——. *Quantum Healing: Exploring the Frontiers of Body, Mind, and Medicine.* New York: Bantam, 1989.

Cousins, Norman. *Head First: The Biology of Hope.* New York: E. P. Dutton, 1989.

Cowens, Deborah and Tom Monte. *A Gift for Healing.* New York: Crown Trade Paperbacks, 1996.

D'Adamo, James. *One Man's Food.* Toronto: Health Thru Herbs Inc., 1980.

Daniel, Alma et al. *Ask Your Angels.* New York: Ballantine Books, 1992.

Davies, Stevan L. *Jesus the Healer.* New York: Continuum, 1995.

de Waal, Esther. *Seeking God: The Way of St. Benedict.* Collegeville, MN: Liturgical Press, 1984.

DelBene, Ron. *The Hunger of the Heart: The Call to Spiritual Growth.* Nashville: Upper Room Books, 1992.

Dewhurst-Maddock, Olivea. *The Book of Sound Therapy: Heal Yourself with Music and Voice.* New York: Simon & Schuster, 1993.

Dong, Paul & Aristide Esser. *Chi Gong: The Ancient Chinese Way to Health.* New York: Paragon House, 1990.

Dossey, Larry. *Healing Words: The Power of Prayer and the Practice of Medicine.* New York: HarperSanFrancisco, 1993.

——. *Prayer is Good Medicine.* San Francisco: HarperCollins, 1996.

Douglas-Klottz, Neil. *Prayers of the Cosmos: Meditations on the Aramaic Words of Jesus.* New York: HarperSanFrancisco, 1990.

Downie, Peter. *Healers at Work.* Kelowna, BC: Northstone, 1996.

Downing, Christine, ed. *Mirrors of the Self: Archetypal Images Shape Your Life.* Los Angeles: Jeremy P. Tarcher, 1991.

Eisenberg, David S. & Thomas L. Wright. *Encounters with Qi.* New York: Viking Penguin, 1987.

Elliot, Clifford. *With Integrity of Heart: Living Values in Changing Times.* New York: Friendship Press, 1991.

Fahrion, S., ed. *Subtle Energies: An Interdisciplinary Journal of Energetic and Informational Interactions.* Golden, CO: ISSSEEM, various issues.

Foster, Richard J. *Coming Home: A Prayer Journal.* New York: HarperCollins, 1994.

——. *Prayer: Finding the Heart's True Home.* New York: HarperSanFrancisco, 1992.

Fox, Matthew & Rupert Sheldrake. *The Physics of Angels: Exploring the Realm Where Science and Spirit Meet.* New York: Harper SanFrancisco, 1996.

Fox, Matthew. *A Spirituality Named Compassion.* New York: HarperSanFrancisco, 1990.

Frankl, Victor. *Man's Search for Meaning.* New York: Pocketbooks, 1988

Friedman, Norman. *Bridging Science and Spirit.* St. Louis, MO: Living Lake Books, 1994.

Gerber, Richard. *Vibrational Medicine. New Choices for Healing Ourselves.* Santa Fe: Bear, 1988.

Goleman, Daniel & Joel Gurin. *Mind/Body Medicine.* New York: Consumer Reports Books, 1993.

Gorsuch, John P. *An Invitation to the Spiritual Journey.* New York: Paulist Press, 1990.

Graham, Billy. *Angels: God's Secret Agents.* Waco, TX: Word Books, 1986.

Green, Elmer & Alyce Green. *Beyond Biofeedback.* Ft. Wayne, TX:
Knoll Publishing, 1989.

Gribbin, John. *Schrödinger's Kittens and the Search for Reality.* Toronto: Little, Brown, 1995.

Haas, Elson M. *Staying Healthy with the Seasons.* Berkeley, CA: Celestial Arts, 1981.

Hanh, Thich Nhat. *Peace Is Every Step: The Path of Mindfulness in Everyday Life.* New York:
Bantam, 1992.

Hahnemann, Samuel. *Organon of Medicine.* New Delhi, India: B. Jain Publishers, 1990.

Harpur, Tom. *For Christ's Sake.* Toronto: Oxford University Press, 1986.

——. *The Uncommon Touch: An Investigation of Spiritual Healing.* Toronto: McClelland &
Stewart, 1994.

Hildegard of Bingen. *Illuminations of Hildegard of Bingen.* Santa Fe, NM: Bear, 1985.

Hover-Kramer, Dorothea. *Healing Touch, A Resource for Health Care Professionals.* Albany, NY:
Delmar, 1996.

Jacobi, Jolande. *The Psychology of C.G. Jung.* London: Yale University Press, 1973.

Jahn, Robert & Brenda J. Dunne. *Margins of Reality: The Role of Consciousness in the Physical
World.* Orlando, FL: Harcourt Brace & Co., 1987.

Johnston, William. *Being in Love: The Practice of Christian Prayer.* San Francisco: Harper &
Row, 1989.

——. *Silent Music: The Science of Meditation.* San Francisco: Harper & Row, 1979.

Joy, W. Brugh. *Joy's Way.* Los Angeles: Jeremy P. Tarcher, 1979.

Jung, Carl G. *Psychology & Religion.* New Haven: Yale University Press, 1966.

——. *Man and His Symbols.* New York: Dell, 1968.

Kaisch, K. *Finding God: A Handbook of Christian Meditation.* New York: Paulist Press, 1994.

Karagulla, Shajica & Dora Van Gelder Kunz. *The Chakras and the Human Energy Fields.* Wheaton,
IL: Theosophical Publishing House, 1989.

Keating, Thomas. *Open Mind, Open Heart: The Contemplative Dimension of the Gospel.* New
York: Continuum, 1995.

Kelsey, Morton. *Healing and Christianity.* New York: Harper & Row, 1973.

——. *The Other Side of Silence: A Guide to Christian Meditation.* New York: Paulist Press, 1976.

Krieger, Dolores. *Accepting Your Power to Heal.* Santa Fe, NM: Bear, 1993.

——. *Living the Therapeutic Touch.* New York: Dodd, Mead, 1987.

——. *Therapeutic Touch: How to Use Your Hands to Help or to Heal.* New York: Prentice Hall, 1986.

Kurtz, Ron. *Body-Centered Psychotherapy: The Hakomi Method.* Mendocino, CA: LifeRhythm, 1990.

Laskow, Leonard. *Healing With Love.* New York: HarperSanFrancisco, 1992.

Lawrence, Brother. *The Practice of the Presence of God.* Garden City, NY: Doubleday, 1977.

Lawrence, Roy. *Christian Healing Rediscovered.* Downers Grove, IL: InterVarsity Press, 1980.

Leadbeater, Charles W. *Man: Visible & Invisible.* Wheaton, IL: Theosophical Publishing House, 1987.

Lingerman, Hal A. *The Healing Energies of Music.* Wheaton, IL: Quest, 1983.

Lowen, Alexander. *Depression and the Body: The Biological Basis of Faith and Reality.*
New York: Penguin, 1972.

MacRae, Janet. *Therapeutic Touch: A Practical Guide.* New York: Alfred A. Knopf, 1996.

Main, John. *Word into Silence.* London: Darton, Longman & Todd, 1985.

Manning, Doug. *Don't Take My Grief Away: What to Do When You Lose a Loved One.* San Francisco: HarperSanFrancisco, 1984.

Martinez, F. Garcia, Julia Trebolle Barrera, & Wilfred G. Watson. *The People of the Dead Sea Scrolls: Their Writings, Beliefs and Practices.* Leiden, The Netherlands: E.J.Brill, 1995.

Michael, Chester & Marie C. Norrisey. *Prayer and Temperament: Prayer Forms for Different Personality Types.* Charlottesville, VA: The Open Door, 1984.

Miller, Robert J., ed. *The Complete Gospels: Annotated Scholars Version.* Sonoma, CA: Polebridge Press, 1994.

Moore, Thomas. *Care of the Soul.* New York: HarperCollins, 1992.

Motoyama, Hiroshi. *Karma and Reincarnation.* New York: Avon, 1992.

Myss, Caroline M. *Anatomy of the Spirit.* New York: Crown, 1996.

Nightingale, Florence. *Suggestions for Thought.* Philadelphia: University of Pennsylvania Press, 1994.

Nodwell, R. Gordon. *A Christian Perspective on Healing.* Toronto: The United Church of Canada, 1977.

North Carolina Center for Healing Touch Publishers. *Healing Touch, Level 1 Notebook.* North Carolina, 1994.

Northrup, Christiane. *Women's Bodies, Women's Wisdom.* New York: Bantam Books, 1994.

Nouwen, Henri J. M. *Behold the Beauty of the Lord: Praying with Icons.* Notre Dame, IN: Ave Maria, 1987

—— *Genesee Diary: Report from a Trappist Monastery.* New York: Image, 1981.

——. *Here and Now: Living in the Spirit.* New York: Crossroads, 1995.

——. *Life of the Beloved: Spiritual Living in a Secular World.* New York: Crossroad, 1992.

——. *The Way of the Heart.* New York: Ballantine, 1981.

——. *The Wounded Healer.* New York: Image Books, 1979.

Oldfield, Harry & Roger Coghill. *The Dark Side of the Brain.* Longmead, Dorset: Element Books, 1988.

Olsen, Kirsten Gottschalk. *The Encyclopedia of Alternative Health Care.* New York: Pocket Books, 1990.

Owen, Robert. *Qualitative Research: The Early Years.* Salem, OR: Grayhaven Books, 1988.

Pagels, Elaine. *The Origin of Satan.* New York: Vintage Books, Random House, 1995.

Paterson, Morton. *Dr. Jesus: A Wholeness Therapy for Our Day.* Hamilton: Self & Olivet United Church, 1993.

Peat, F. David. *Infinite Potential: The Life & Times of David Bohm.* Don Mills: Addison-Wesley Publishing, 1997.

Peck, M. Scott. *Further Along the Road Less Traveled.* New York: Simon and Schuster, 1993.

——. *People of the Lie.* New York: Simon & Schuster, 1983.

Penrose, Roger. *Shadows of the Mind*. New York: Oxford University Press, 1994.

——. *The Emperor's New Mind*. New York: Oxford University Press, 1989.

Pomeranz, B., & G. Stux. *Acupuncture: Textbook and Atlas*. New York: Springer-Verlag, 1987.

Postema, Donald. *Space for God: The Study and Practice of Prayer and Spirituality*. Grand Rapids: CRC Publications, 1983.

Puryear, Herbert B. *Why Jesus Taught Reincarnation: A Better News Gospel*. Scottsdale, AZ: New Paradigm Press, 1992.

Roth, Nancy. *The Breath of God. An Approach to Prayer*. Cambridge, MA: Cowley, 1990.

Rubik, Beverly, ed. *The Interrelationship between Mind & Matter*. Philadelphia: Center for Frontier Sciences, 1992.

Rupp, Joyce. *May I Have This Dance?* Notre Dame, IN: Ave Maria Press, 1992.

——. *The Star in My Heart: Experiencing Sophia, Inner Wisdom*. San Diego: LuraMedia, 1990

Russell, Peter. *The Brain Book: Application of Brain Research to Self-improvement*. New York: Penguin, 1979.

Saint John of the Cross. *Dark Night of the Soul*. New York: Doubleday, 1959.

Saint Teresa of Avila. *Interior Castle*. Garden City, NY: Doubleday, 1961.

Sanford, Agnes. *The Healing Gifts of the Spirit*. Philadelphia: J.B.Lippincott, 1966.

——. *The Healing Light*. Plainfield, NJ: MacAlester Park Pub., 1976.

——. *The Healing Power of the Bible*. New York: J.B. Lippincott, 1977.

——. *The Healing Touch of God*. Toronto: Ballantine, 1983.

Sanford, John A. *Healing and Wholeness*. New York: Paulist Press, 1977.

——. *Healing Body and Soul*. Louisville: Westminster/John Knox, 1992.

Savary, Louis M., and Patricia H. Berne. *Kything: The Art of Spiritual Presence*. Mahwah, NJ: Paulist Press, 1988.

Schroeder, Celeste Snowber. *Embodied Prayer*. Liguori, MI: Triumph Books, 1994.

Schwarz, Jack. *Human Energy Systems*. New York: Viking Penguin, 1980.

——. *Voluntary Controls*. Toronto: Penguin Books (Arkara), 1978 .

Shapiro, Debbie. *The Body-Mind Workbook*. Shaftesbury, Dorset: Element Books Ltd., 1990.

Shealy, C. Norman, and Caroline M. Myss. *The Creation of Health*. Walpole, NH: Stillpoint Publishing, 1988.

Sheldrake, Rupert. *A New Science of Life: The Hypothesis of Formative Creation*. Los Angeles: J. P. Tarcher, 1981.

Stahl, Carolyn. *Opening to God: Guided Imagery Meditation on Scripture*. Nashville: The Upper Room, 1977.

Stringfellow, William. *Instead of Death*. New York: Seabury, 1963.

——. *A Private and Public Faith*. Grand Rapids, MI: Wm. B. Eerdmans, 1962.

Talbot, Michael. *The Holographic Universe*. New York: HarperCollins, 1991.

Tart, Charles T. *Altered States of Consciousness*. New York: HarperCollins, 1990.

Taylor, James. *Sin: A New Understanding of Virtue and Vice*. Kelowna, BC: Northstone, 1997.

Thomas, Zach. *Healing Touch: The Church's Forgotten Language.* Louisville: Westminster/John Knox Press, 1994.

Thompson, Marjorie J. *Soul Feast: An Invitation to the Christian Spiritual Feast.* Louisville: Westminster/John Knox, 1995.

Ulanov, Ann, and Barry Ulanov. *Primary Speech: A Psychology of Prayer.* Atlanta: John Knox, 1982.

Vithoulkas, George. *The Science of Homeopathy: The Laws and Principles of Cure.* New York: Grove Atlantic, 1980.

Wagner, James K. *An Adventure in Healing and Wholeness.* Nashville: Upper Room, 1993.

——. *Blessed to Be a Blessing.* Nashville: Upper Room, 1980.

Waldrop, M. Mitchell. *Complexity: The Emerging Science at the Edge of Order.* New York: Simon & Schuster, 1992.

Watson, Lyall. *Supernature II.* Great Britain: Hodder & Stoughton, 1973.

——. *The Nature of Things: The Secret Life of Inanimate Objects.* Great Britain: Hodder & Stoughton, 1990.

——. *The Dreams of Dragons: and Other Writings on the Edge of Natural History.* Rochester, Vermont: Destiny Books, 1992.

Weatherhead, Leslie D. *The Case for Reincarnation.* London, England: City Temple, 1971.

Weiss, Bernard L. *Many Lives, Many Masters.* New York: Simon & Schuster, 1988.

Westberg, Grainger E. *The Parish Nurse.* Minneapolis: Augsburg, 1990.

Weston, Walter L. *Pray Well: A Holistic Guide to Health and Renewal.* Wadsworth, OH: Transitions Press, 1994.

Wilbur, K. *The Spectrum of Consciousness.* Wheaton, IL: Quest, 1993.

Worrall, Ambrose & Olga Worrall. *The Gift of Healing.* New York: Harper & Row, 1965.

Wuellner, Flora Slosson. *Prayer, Stress and our Inner Wounds.* Nashville: Upper Room, 1985.

——. *Heart of Healing, Heart of Light.* Nashville: Upper Room Books, 1992.

——. *Prayer and our Bodies.* Nashville: Upper Room, 1993.

——. *Release.* Nashville: Upper Room Books, 1996.